Partnerships for Health
and Human Service Nonprofits

Tine Hansen-Turton, MGA, JD, FCPP, FAAN, is the chief strategy officer of Public Health Management Corporation (PHMC), where she develops and supports PHMC's overall strategy and leads partnership development around new and emerging business opportunities. She works across the organization, but specifically oversees Management Services and the Research and Evaluation Group. She also manages organizational development and learning, regional emergency preparedness services, and mergers and affiliations, as well as the trade associations the National Nursing Centers Consortium and the Convenient Care Association. She is nationally known for her development and policy systems change work with nurse-led care as well as for expanding access to care for millions through convenient care (retail) clinics.

Richard J. Cohen, PhD, FACHE, is recognized nationally as an authority in the public health management arena. He is the chief executive officer (CEO) of Public Health Management Corporation (PHMC), where he leads 1,400 employees, more than 250 public health programs, and numerous subsidiary organizations that have become affiliated with PHMC during more than 20 years of mergers and acquisitions. Under his watch, the organization has expanded exponentially and continues to grow, with a current operating budget of approximately $180 million. Dr. Cohen has devoted his professional life to the needs of Philadelphia and the surrounding region while playing a critical role at a national level as well.

Nicholas D. Torres, MEd, is a cofounder of the *Philadelphia Social Innovations Journal*. He also serves as a senior fellow for Public/Private Ventures and is the president of Education-Plus, Inc., where he scales 9 to 14 college-access and completion models for low-income students, school-based health centers, and quality education interventions for specialized populations via blended learning models.

Partnerships for Health and Human Service Nonprofits

From Collaborations to Mergers

Tine Hansen-Turton, MGA, JD, FCPP, FAAN
Richard J. Cohen, PhD, FACHE
Nicholas D. Torres, MEd

Editors

SPRINGER PUBLISHING COMPANY
NEW YORK

Springer Publishing Company, LLC
11 West 42nd Street
New York, NY 10036
www.springerpub.com

Acquisitions Editor: Stephanie Drew
Production Editor: Michael O'Connor
Composition: Newgen Knowledge Works

ISBN: 978-0-8261-2806-5
e-book ISBN: 978-0-8261-2808-9

14 15 16 17 18/ 5 4 3 2 1

Library of Congress Cataloging-in-Publication Data
Partnerships for health and human service nonprofits : from collaborations to mergers / [edited by] Tine Hansen-Turton, Richard J. Cohen, Nicholas D. Torres.
    p. ; cm.
Includes bibliographical references.
ISBN 978-0-8261-2806-5 — ISBN 978-0-8261-2808-9 (e-book)
    I. Hansen-Turton, Tine, editor. II. Cohen, Richard J. (President and CEO of the Philadelphia Health Management Corporation), editor. III. Torres, Nicholas D., editor.
    [DNLM: 1. Health Care Sector—organization & administration—Pennsylvania. 2. Health Facility Merger—Pennsylvania. 3. Health Policy—Pennsylvania. 4. Organizational Case Studies—Pennsylvania. 5. Organizations, Nonprofit—Pennsylvania. W 74 AP4]
    RA407.4.P4
    362.109748—dc23   2014034254

Printed in the United States of America by McNaughton & Gunn.

Contents

Contributors

Judith Bernstein-Baker, Esq., MSW, JD
Executive Director
HIAS Pennsylvania
Philadelphia, PA

Allison F. Book, MPA
Lawrenceville, NJ

William P. Brown, Jr., MS, BS
President and CEO
Advanced Living Communities
Lansdale, PA

Jacob Cavallo, BA
Urban Affairs Coalition
Philadelphia, PA

Richard J. Cohen, PhD, FACHE
Chief Executive Officer
Public Health Management
    Corporation
Philadelphia, PA

Carl M. Coyle, MSW
Chief Executive Officer
Liberty Resources, Inc.
Chief Executive Officer
MESA Inc
Syracuse, NY

Ashley Del Bianco, MSEd., MPA
Program Director
City of Philadelphia Office of
    Innovation and Technology
Philadelphia, PA

Tivoni Devor, MBA
Manager of Partnerships and
    Outreach
Urban Affairs Coalition
Philadelphia, PA

Patricia Hampson Eget, PhD
Assistant Director of Corporate and
    Foundation Relations
Saint Joseph's University
Philadelphia, PA

J. Kevin Fee, BA
President
Angler West Consultants Inc.
Doylestown, PA

Robert M. Gallagher, MS
Chief Executive Officer
North Penn YMCA
Colmar, PA

Will Gonzalez, JD
Executive Director
Ceiba
Philadelphia, PA

**Tine Hansen-Turton, MGA, JD,
    FCPP, FAAN**
Chief Strategy Officer
Public Health Management
    Corporation
Chief Executive Officer
National Nursing Centers Consortium
Philadelphia, PA

Taz Hussein, MBA
Partner
The Bridgespan Group
Boston, MA

Russell Johnson, MSW
President and Chief Executive
    Officer
North Penn Community Health
    Foundation
Colmar, PA

Natasha Keleman, MSS
Executive Director
Pennsylvania Immigration and
    Citizenship Coalition
Philadelphia, PA

Annette Mattei, MPA/MSES
Principal
Metro Metrics, LLC
Philadelphia, PA

Joan C. Mazzotti, JD
Executive Director
Philadelphia Futures
Philadelphia, PA

Thomas A. McLaughlin, MBA, MS
Principal
McLaughlin & Associates
Adjunct Lecturer
Heller School at Brandeis University
Andover, MA

Katie Smith Milway, BA, MBA
Partner
Head of Knowledge
The Bridgespan Group
Boston, MA

James Moss, MS
Academic Engagement Coordinator
University of Pennsylvania Museum
    of Archaeology and Anthropology
Philadelphia, PA

Ann O'Brien, MSS, MLSP, MBA
Chief Executive Officer
Montgomery Early Learning Centers
Narberth, PA

Maria Orozco, BA, MA
Manager
The Bridgespan Group
New York, NY

Arun Prabhakaran, BA
Vice President and Chief External
    Affairs Officer
Urban Affairs Coalition
Philadelphia, PA

Kate Rivera, BA
Project Director
Urban Affairs Coalition
Philadelphia, PA

Arianne Sellers, MPA , BA
Operations Manager
Innovations Home Care
West Conshohocken, PA

Gretchen Shanfeld, MPH
Refugee Health Coordinator
Nationalities Service Center
Philadelphia, PA

Ashley Tobin, MPA
Work Better Consulting
Turning Points for Children
Philadelphia, PA

Nicholas D. Torres, MEd
President
Education-Plus, Inc.,
Bryn Mawr, PA

Kathy Wellbank, MSS, LSW
Program Director
Interim House
Philadelphia, PA

Introduction

Katie Smith Milway and Maria Orozco

MERGERS AND COLLABORATIONS: FINDING THE RIGHT MODEL

Consider this true story: Two nonprofits, leaders in their field, saw tremendous mission and program synergies, which they tested through a variety of collaborations. Confident that a full merger could scale their impact, they announced their intent, formed a merger committee across top leadership, and began formulating program, funding, and branding strategies. Then they hit a barrier: Despite apparent program advantages and the potential to raise more money as a merged organization, the time and cost of integrating financial, human resource, and information systems was too high. They jointly agreed to abandon the deal.

No question, mergers and collaborations can strengthen a field—they can more rapidly scale a proven approach to employing disaffected youth, preventing teen pregnancy, or expanding environmental conservation—more than building out programs site by site. These partnerships can add new capabilities and opportunities to access more clients, and they can streamline operations. They can also stem needless reinvention. But as is equally clear from our opening tale, the process of finding the right model for combining forces is not simple, even when the advantages seem overwhelmingly obvious.

In the spring of 2014, Bridgespan, La Piana Consulting, The Lodestar Foundation, and The Catalyst Fund for Nonprofits joined forces to explore "Mergers That Make a Difference," via a microsite on Bridgespan.org of cases and blogs (www.bridgespan.org/mergers-and-collaborations). As part of our exploration, we asked executives who had successfully led mergers that increased their organizations' impact to share how they overcame challenges, and to suggest how peers considering mergers could lessen the risk of failure. Their responses converged on four key pieces of advice, relevant to a range of collaborations:

Think Mission Versus Organization

Rachel Haag, former CEO of Boston's AIDS Action Committee (AAC), completed three mergers on behalf of AAC in 4 years, most recently between AAC and Fenway Health. She said the key in each was for leaders to check egos at the door and focus on future missions, not on current organizations or even on their own jobs, a sentiment echoed by other bloggers in the series. "There is just no place for egos in nonprofit mergers," Haag said. "Instead of thinking, 'How does this merger affect me?' board members and senior staff must evaluate every merger-related decision by asking, 'How does this enhance our organization's ability to meet its mission?' At AAC, we developed a set of criteria that required us to document how a merger would improve client quality of care, ensure organizational sustainability, and allow us to continue to tackle the root causes of HIV/AIDS." Similarly, collaborations short of merging can call for parties to clarify decision-making roles and relinquish power to be effective. Said Haag, "It was paramount that our mission was preserved; organizational integrity or the future role of board members or senior staff was secondary."

Match Merger (or Collaboration) Funding to True Costs

Merger due diligence and integration can create high one-time costs, and merger funders need to cover them. But many funders fail to acknowledge the true costs of forging a union, from back-office integration to rebranding. For example, Linda Johanek, CEO of the Domestic

Violence & Child Advocacy Center (DVCAC) in Cleveland discussed the ongoing costs of rebranding. "One year after the Domestic Violence Center and the Bellflower Center for Prevention of Child Abuse changed names (to become DVCAC), donations dropped twenty-five percent," said Johanek. "Two years after the merger, we continue to rebrand and search for the money to do so." Good Shepherd estimated that its integration of a neighborhood services acquisition in 2012 took two years and $570,000, not including staff time or pro bono legal assistance. Funder John MacIntosh of Seachange Capital Partners estimated that a three-way charter school merger that Seachange backed cost $250,000 and was worth every penny. Yet too often, funders are not aligned. Says Johanek: "One funder denied our request to help with merger-associated costs, advising that we 'use the money [we were] saving [through the merger] to fund the transition.'...That funder clearly didn't understand there are many associated costs that continue past the signing of a merger...." Collaborations, too, can take a significant investment of leadership and line-staff time, and collaborators need to count those costs. Johanek concluded, "I call upon all funders to have a long-term vision when a newly merged agency is seeking to create long-term benefits."

Prioritize Cultural Due Diligence

Sister Paulette LoMonaco, executive director of Good Shepherd Services (GSS), and GSS associate executive director Laurie Williams pointed to the primacy of cultural due diligence when assessing acquisitions. Meanwhile, Stephen Payne, executive director of the recently merged Oakland East Bay Symphony, spoke of the importance of building a new culture. The crystal clear message: When collaborating in any way, pay attention to culture. In a 2009 Bridgespan survey titled "Finding Leaders for America's Nonprofits," out of 433 nonprofit leaders, three-quarters ranked cultural fit as a make-or-break quality for incoming nonprofit leaders. It stands to reason that the stakes are much higher when a collaboration or merger brings in multiple leaders. Says Sr. Paulette, "[We] require what we call *cultural due diligence*, which we define as spending the time, energy, and money to carefully plan how we will incorporate staff from the acquired entities into the culture of Good Shepherd Services. Of course, we learned about [its] importance ... the hard way."

Make Staff the Architects of Integration

Elisabeth Babcock, executive director of Crittenton Women's Union (CWU), agrees that board and staff egos can be the greatest barriers to strategic unions. But she credits the legacy boards of CWU with avoiding these pitfalls by deputizing senior staff to create a blueprint for the merger. Says Babcock: "Tap your senior staff and trust their ability to provide valuable analysis on the potential upsides and roadblocks of this type of transition. In the case of Crittenton Women's Union, it was staff at both legacy organizations who were able to envision a more streamlined and strategic organization that could propel a greater number of low-income women to economic independence." Good Shepherd has used merger integration assignments as a form of senior staff leadership development. The Cancer Support Community born of the merger of The Wellness Community and Gilda's Club Worldwide developed a transition leadership committee comprising board members and staff from the merging organizations and their affiliates; from the beginning, the affiliates were an integral part of the decision-making process. In any form of collaboration, staff closest to the action will have perspective on how the pieces best fit together to achieve joint goals.

To these four messages, we would like to add one more piece of advice, which Babcock passed on while describing the range of tactics her organization has used to amplify its programs and resources on behalf of the women and children it serves. Always look for the least complicated form of collaboration to achieve the impact you seek. Sometimes, this will call for merging, as her organization did. But there are also many simpler ways for nonprofits to collaborate—from sharing best practices to loose coalitions for advocacy to joint ventures to allow for sharing and managing assets to colocating to share services.

In fact, we believe there is a spectrum of options that nonprofits can use to align with others and achieve greater impact:

- Associations
  A group of organizations voluntarily combines forces to accomplish a purpose over time

Includes coalitions (e.g., The Green Justice Coalition), collaboratives (e.g., Strive), and communities of practice (e.g., the Lodestar Collaboration Prize)

- Joint Programming
  A contractual programmatic undertaking of two or more entities without actual legal incorporation (e.g., Career Family Opportunity Cambridge, CWU, Cambridge Housing Authority)
- Shared Administrative Services
  Jointly hiring a third party or agreeing to share an existing resource to provide services such as accounting, marketing, IT, or office space to consolidate administrative functions (e.g., the colocation and cobranding of AARP and Experience Corps)
- Mergers
  Two organizations combine into one. This can be accomplished through legal affiliate or subsidiary structures, integrating one organization into another, or creating a new entity (e.g., the Hillside Family of Agencies affiliates; the merging and rebranding of The Wellness Community and Gilda's Club Worldwide into the Cancer Support Community).

The journey along the collaboration-to-merger spectrum (Figure I.1) starts by being clear about the impact you seek to create and evaluating the capabilities, clients, and scale you will need to achieve it. Only then consider whether it makes most sense to invest to *build* these assets, to collaborate and *borrow* them, or to acquire or *buy* them through a merger. When there is not a clear rationale or through line to impact, saying no to a merger or collaboration may be the best answer.

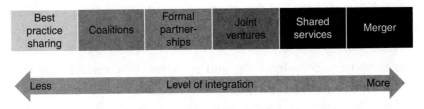

FIGURE I.1 The collaboration-to-merger spectrum.

- Question 1: What impact do we seek to create?
- Question 2: What capabilities, clients, and scale do we need to create it?
- Question 3: Should we build, borrow, or buy to get there?

If your analysis of needs, of providers, and of the economics of service delivery leads you to consider the borrow or buy options, there is another series of questions: How can you find the right partner for a merger or collaboration? Fund the true cost of due diligence and integration? And, if you buy, how can you create a blueprint for integration that carefully considers three traps that too often sink even strategically aligned mergers: blending boards, blending staff, and blending brands? Asking and answering these questions may lead you to a different place on the collaboration spectrum.

For example, Clyde Comstock, chief operating officer at the Hillside Family of Agencies in New York, which grew through nine acquisitions, has learned to create other forms of collaboration when talks about merging board or brand will not work. One approach is to construct a legal affiliate relationship, whereby a large organization that wants to partner without losing its identity can keep its brand, its 501(c)(3) status, and a board appointed by Hillside to govern its operations, essentially as a subsidiary within the parent organization. "As parent, we appoint the board on each of the affiliate organizations using a nominating committee with representation from all the boards [of all our affiliates]." Some member of an affiliate's board might plug into the parent's board, by serving on Hillside's overarching finance committee or other task force. Looser affiliate relationships also are possible (for more on affiliate relationships, see Charity Lawyer at http://charitylawyerblog.com/2011/02/01/creating-nonprofit-chapters-and-affiliates). Regardless of construct, Hillside works hard to preserve the unique identity of each partner. "If it's a merger, acquired organizations still keep their identity as [sub-brands]. We've been focused on all the options."

The United States has nearly 40 nonprofits per zip code, based on data from the Urban Institute, and many of their leaders, like those in our opening story, see potential value in consolidation. Recent Bridgespan research found that 20% of nonprofit leaders were considering mergers as part of their strategy, and more than 60% were engaging in some form of collaboration. So it is not surprising that questions of when and how to pursue mergers and collaborations are being asked by social innovators, whatever their organization's legal structure or stage of development.

Nor should it be surprising that there will never be one right answer to these questions. Every alternative will carry trade-offs—in autonomy, risk, and the investments of time, money, and talent required. Coalitions that engage many organizations, for example, may have difficulty creating significant, meaningful change. Partnerships can be strengthened through formal memos of understanding and processes, but without integration, there is no guarantee the relationship will continue. Shared services are likely to require significant legal and operational alignment, meaning cost, revenue, and other benefits may not materialize in the short term.

When planning collaborations, it is critical to address the pros and cons of each structure. Ultimately, of course, the right approach will depend on the goals of the collaboration and the parties involved.

We hope you learn as much from these chapters as we have.

1

Partnership Introduction and Nonprofits in the 21st Century

Tine Hansen-Turton, Nicholas D. Torres, and Richard J. Cohen

THE NONPROFIT SECTOR IN THE 21ST CENTURY

Charitable giving and the provision of services for the needy without expectation of remuneration have been a part of this country's social fabric since America's inception (Glavin, 2011). According to the Urban Institute's National Center for Charitable Statistics, there are currently 1,574,674 tax-exempt organizations across the country (Urban Institute, n.d.): 959,698 charitable organizations, 100,337 private foundations, and 514,639 "other" organizations, which encompass, among a broad array of entities, chambers of commerce and professional and fraternal associations. By far, 501(c)(3) organizations are the majority of nonprofits in the United States. These can include both public charities and private foundations (Urban Institute, 2008). The category of private charities is made up of very large organizations, such as hospitals, academic institutions, and museums, as well as small organizations, including community theaters and neighborhood groups. Private foundations structured as 501(c)(3)s include both grant-making and operating foundations.

1

The impact of the nonprofit sector on the U.S. economy is substantial (Glavin, 2011). In 2009, nonprofits accounted for 5.4% of the gross domestic product (GDP) and 9% of the total wages and salaries paid nationally. Total expenses and revenues for all public charities in the United States in 2009 were $1.40 trillion and $1.41 trillion, respectively. The majority of public charities' revenues (76%) came from program service revenue, including government fees and contracts. The balance of the revenues was attributable to contributions and gifts, government grants (22%), and other sources including dues, rental income, special event income, and the transfer of goods (11%). Total assets held by U.S. public charities in 2009 totaled $2.56 trillion. These numbers have been buoyed by the growth within the sector itself—the number of nonprofits increased by 25% between 2001 and 2011 (Urban Institute, 2012).

There is also a meaningful indirect economic and social benefit from the nonprofit sector in terms of the rate of private charitable giving and the number of volunteers and volunteer hours contributed. In 2010, total charitable giving by individuals, corporations, and foundations amounted to $290.89 billion (Glavin, 2011). Of that total, $211.77 billion accrued from individual giving. More than a quarter of Americans older than 16 years—approximately 26.3%—volunteered time for or through a nonprofit organization over the course of the period from 2009 to 2010. A report from the Urban Institute concluded that in 2006, nonprofits benefited from a total of 12.9 billion volunteer hours, which equates with 7.6 million full-time employees, at a wage equivalence value of $215.6 billion (Blackwood, Wing, & Pollak, 2008).

The Changing World for Nonprofits

Charles Darwin once said, "It is not the strongest of the species that survives, nor the most intelligent that survives. It is the one that is the most adaptable to change." In the human service industry, the for-profit sector has adapted adroitly to the current trends of budget cutting and privatization of government services through third-party contracts. Although they have been busy consolidating, the 1.6 million (and counting) nonprofit organizations as a whole remain more fragmented, and their abilities to change remain hampered by archaic business structures and advocacy implementation.

In today's environment, we encounter strategic partnerships every day. The impossible becomes possible when a partnership is formed. The nonprofit world is changing, and the future success of the more than 1.6 million nonprofits will be defined and dominated by strategic alignments and partnerships. Funders at all levels are pushing strategic alliances. Innovation that creates social change and impact requires us to abandon our silos and fears and learn to create new partnerships.

In this book, the reader will learn from national leaders and experts about the critical roles strategic alignments and partnerships play in advancing the nonprofit social sector and its impact. The chapters range from successful community grassroots collaborations to full-blown mergers. Each chapter focuses not only on the formation of the strategic partnership but also on the courage— and the risks—it took to create the new entity and have greater impact.

The main partners in this book have been the *Philadelphia Social Innovations Journal* and the Public Health Management Corporation. Other partners include: the Public Health Fund, United Way of Greater Philadelphia and Southern New Jersey, and The Philadelphia Foundation. Throughout this book, readers will learn how health and human service and the general nonprofit sector are partnering. It is a guide based on the lessons learned from many national organizations. Specifically, this book discusses how these organizations, by deploying strategies and having senior leaders in strategy roles, showed that nonprofits can be:

- More agile in adjusting to change
- More data driven in making decisions
- Better positioned to partner
- Better able to innovate in ways that have meaningful impact on reducing poverty throughout America and beyond

Through case studies of nonprofits, including lessons learned, this book will share a new depth of understanding about the role of strategic partnerships at all levels, including knowledge of the tools and methods that have the greatest potential to enhance successful partnerships, mergers, and alliances.

With authors from a variety of national nonprofits and from practitioners in the field, *Partnerships for Health and Human Service Nonprofits: From Collaborations to Mergers* promises to be the first and most comprehensive book on creating meaningful, long-term, and successful partnerships in the nonprofit sector.

At the end of the book, readers will be able to:

- Understand nonprofits' need to begin thinking strategically about consolidations and partnerships to keep their doors open and to grow and scale
- Understand the various partnership models:

    Collaboration: Includes information sharing, program coordination, and joint planning. Organizations involved in collaboration remain independent, with full decision-making power.

    Administrative consolidation: Typically aimed at increasing efficiency; includes formal agreements for contracting, exchanging, or sharing services. Organizations involved in administrative consolidations share decision-making powers.

    Joint programming: A restructuring whereby multiple organizations share the launch and management of one or more programs. Organizations involved in joint programming share decision-making powers for that program while maintaining their independence in managing their own programs.

    Corporate mergers and acquisitions: Includes full integration of all programmatic assets and administrative functions.

- Understand the challenges and opportunities with all types of partnerships
- Recognize the challenges and opportunities for partnering within the health and human service sector
- Discuss how to use partnerships to improve organizational capacity and infrastructure
- Understand how to use data to drive change and impact
- Recognize the need for and ways to align services through partnerships to achieve collective impact
- Understand how to deploy strategy to create purposeful partnerships
- Learn how to implement a successful partnership

THE PURPOSE AND AUDIENCE FOR THIS BOOK

The inspiration for this book grew out of a special edition of the *Philadelphia Social Innovations Journal* in the winter of 2013 in which dozens of regional and national leaders wrote about their experiences with the variety of partnership options and came together to discuss them in February 2013 in Philadelphia. The online journal edition and launch event were a huge success, with more than 300 nonprofit leaders in the room who all wanted to understand the spectrum of partnerships, how to do partnerships themselves, and what lessons others had learned.

This book will serve to fill in the knowledge gap about partnership strategies for leaders, managers, practitioners, students, faculty members, providers, and other general professionals in the nonprofit sector, including health and human service and education, and those who are interested in, working in, or teaching in the nonprofit sector.

CHAPTER OVERVIEWS

This first chapter reviews the state of the nonprofit social sector in the 21st century, provides a historical perspective of the sector's development in the United States, and considers its size and the legal framework in which it operates. Below is a brief summary of each chapter that follows. The chapters are organized according to the Bridgespan Group's framework for partnering:

- Best practice sharing
- Collaborations/coalitions
- Formal partnerships
- Joint ventures
- Shared services
- Mergers and affiliations
- Strategies, tips, and legal documents for partnering

Chapter 1—Partnership Introduction and Nonprofits in the 21st Century: Chapter 1 introduces the overall concept of the book. It gives an overview of the health, status, and contributions of nonprofits in the United States and discusses how the sector going forward must be more open to and adept at strategic partnerships if it hopes to maintain and expand its impact on social services in America.

Chapter 2—The Emerging Market for Nonprofit Control: Business Model Implications: Part 1 of this chapter explores the current face of the human service industry in the context of the Great Recession and the ongoing economic downturn. Specifically, the first part looks at the current business models that govern both for-profits and nonprofits, and follows up with what a new health nonprofit business structure model can and should look like, particularly in the context of an overall weakened U.S. economy, and the consequent challenges that both for-profit and nonprofit entities are encountering. The second part also addresses the seeming conflicts and apparent challenges between nonprofit and for-profit human service providers, including nonprofits' difficulties in competing with for-profits' lobbying and other abilities to influence governments. Both sections emphasize that the nonprofit human service industry's best opportunities to remain effective and impactful in the sector lie in their overall willingness to accept more "corporate" business strategies, including mergers, acquisitions, and other types of collaborations as well as restructuring, in order to take better advantage of the opportunities that for-profit entities have in expanding their roles in the human service sector.

Chapter 3—Identifying the Right Partnership Strategy: This chapter combines several recent articles by nationally renowned consultant Tom McLaughlin on choosing an appropriate collaboration strategy for your organization. The author discusses partnerships, alliances, subsidiaries—and their differences—and concludes that ultimately there are only two fundamental structures to consider: contractual or corporate restructuring. He also shares the importance of utilizing management contracts, to confirm the relationship between the organization and the executive leadership, during partnership processes, and he spells out the necessary components for ideal contracts.

Chapter 4—Building a Culture of Collaboration: Chapter 4 offers case studies of a number of examples of successful partnerships and collaborations taking place around Philadelphia in the past several years. Partnerships have successfully tackled local issues such as bridging the broad digital divide between the city's technology "haves" and "have-nots" and helping undocumented immigrant youth in Philadelphia take advantage of President Obama's recently passed Deferred Action for Childhood Arrivals program. The chapter finishes with a look at just how nonprofits can take advantage of collaboration opportunities to reduce redundancies, expand effective impacts, and even increase revenues.

Chapter 5—Collaboration Case Studies: Chapter 5 looks at more examples of successful collaborations, highlighting an innovative partnership between the YMCA of the USA and UnitedHealth Group (UHG), a national insurer, to fund the YMCA to provide services through its diabetes prevention program to UHG customers nationwide. Other successful partnerships discussed are the alliance between two Philadelphia nonprofits that separately served the local Asian American community in diverse ways and joined forces to unify and expand their services and another innovative Montgomery County, Pennsylvania, collaboration project to colocate four county nonprofits on one shared campus, sharing facilities and resources to, again, reduce redundancies, expand service provision, and more effectively use financial resources.

Chapter 6—Joint Ventures in the Social Sector: In this chapter, the authors present a framework of three styles of partnership: marriage, parent/child, and prenuptial. Brief case studies are presented of four joint ventures in Philadelphia, two of which were sustained and two of which dissolved, and the authors conclude that only a marriage-style partnership has the best chance of being sustainable in the long run.

Chapter 7—Administrative Consolidations, Administrative Services Organizations, and Joint Programming: Chapter 7 looks at partnerships from the administrative perspective, how back-office operations are managed following affiliations and other partnership efforts. Highlighted are shared-service organizations, which contract with individual agencies to assess their back-office (human resources, bookkeeping, accounting, etc.) needs and conduct them out of house, leaving the organizations themselves to dedicate their staff and financial resources to their programs and missions.

Chapter 8—Merger Myths: In Chapter 8, Tom McLaughlin, noted national nonprofit strategist with a special emphasis on mergers, acquisitions, and other partnerships, gives an overview of the myths that tend to surround the idea of mergers and keep people from pursuing them. Notable are the fear of job losses and the belief that mergers will save the resulting organization money compared to the expenditures of the previously independent organizations. The chapter also takes a look at one successful partnership's thorough due diligence process, dedicated behind-the-scene negotiations, and ultimate success through perseverance and a mutual commitment to the resulting organization's mission.

Chapter 9—Merger Case Studies: Chapter 9 offers a selection of successful merger case studies, beginning with how Public Health Management Corporation manages the partnerships it enters into. Success stories include the incorporation of a traumatic brain injury program into a regional rehabilitation center that was failing, the creation of United Way of Greater Philadelphia and Southern New Jersey through the merger of seven different United Ways, and the merger of two Philadelphia organizations that were each dedicated to providing low-income, high-achieving high-school students with the support necessary to see them pursue and achieve college and careers.

Chapter 10—Strategies, Tips, and Legal Partnership Documents: Chapter 10 provides the toolkit containing some of the documents that organizations interested in pursuing a partnership will likely need during the process. Materials include sample management and affiliation agreements, a sample letter to a state attorney general requesting approval of the partnership, and a thorough due diligence checklist.

REFERENCES

Blackwood, A., Wing, K. T., & Pollak, T. H. (2008). *The nonprofit sector in brief: Facts and figures from the nonprofit Almanac 2008: Public charities, giving, and volunteering.* Washington, DC: The Urban Institute. Retrieved from www.urban.org/UploadedPDF/411664_facts_and_figures.pdf

Glavin, R. (2011). The role of nonprofits in American life. In D. R. Heyman (Ed.), *Nonprofit management 101: A complete and practical guide for leaders and professionals* (pp. 5–20). San Francisco, CA: Jossey-Bass.

The Urban Institute. (n.d.). *Quick facts about nonprofits.* Washington, DC: National Center for Charitable Statistics. Retrieved from www.nccs.urban.org/statistics/quickfacts.cfm

The Urban Institute. (2008). *Nonprofit organizations: Overview.* Washington, DC: National Center for Charitable Statistics. Retrieved from www.nccsdataweb.urban.org/nonprofit-overview.html

The Urban Institute. (2012). *Research area: Nonprofit sector.* Washington, DC: National Center for Charitable Statistics. Retrieved from www.urban.org/nonprofits/more.cfm

2

The Emerging Market for Nonprofit Control: Business Model Implications

J. Kevin Fee and Arianne Sellers

EDITORS' OVERVIEW

As this chapter will reveal, the nonprofit sector has not had a strong history of strategic partnerships; as such, examples of formal best practices can be difficult to come by. Later chapters, in fact, discuss both successes and failures in affiliation and collaboration techniques among nonprofits, including details on what the parties involved found to be the most valuable or most problematic aspects of the affiliations. But this chapter first gives an overview of what has been and is versus what could be in the business models for both the nonprofit and the for-profit sectors, with the aim of, let us say, shaking things up in the nonprofit world's business-as-usual model. Mr. Fee offers a suggestion for how nonprofits can better compete and serve their missions by presenting a potential new nonprofit-sector business model. Ms. Sellers shares an overview of the differences in structure between for-profit and nonprofit business entities, and highlights how nonprofits can take some of the more effective aspects of for-profit operations and reinvigorate the industry to use its existing resources to do more with less, and to turn less into more.

THE STATE OF THE NONPROFIT INDUSTRY

J. Kevin Fee

The Great Recession and its aftermath have adversely impacted the operations of nonprofit organizations (Nonprofit Finance Fund, 2011) at the very time that demand for services has been increasing. This circumstance and recognition that the current economic downturn may be of extended duration have prompted renewed discussion of how nonprofit organizations might create economies of scale through innovative business combinations.

While the scale of individual nonprofit organizations may have little relevance to solving some social problems (Kania & Kramer, 2011), it is an important and timely consideration in the evolution of the fragmented behavioral health and social services industry. Changes in the industry's operating environment are harbingers of rapid consolidation, especially within the disjointed nonprofit provider sector. These changes include differences in the ways services are delivered and financed, shifts in legislation and regulation, consumer preferences, and provider leadership. This new environment presents the typical undercapitalized nonprofit human service provider with the need to provide an expanded array of often technology-enabled services, under an unfamiliar, at-risk contractual arrangement, frequently during a period of executive transition. These challenges have been exacerbated by the economic downturn, which has given rise to an intense provider rivalry encouraged by payers seeking to reduce costs.

As in other industries, these circumstances encourage industry consolidation and hence, the evolution of a market for corporate control. Yet very few nonprofit organizations possess the capital, competences, or experience required to consolidate. Furthermore, few are in a position to develop the required capabilities due to the structural and other barriers associated with traditional nonprofit business models. These models have historically been program centric and differentiated primarily as a consequence of their sizes, as measured by annual revenues.

Clearly, a new business model is needed for the new paradigm, one that enables nonprofit organizations to adapt to the industry's greater demands and the emerging market for corporate control without sacrificing core values. The goals of the new business model will be rapid growth supported by improved governance and new mechanisms for accumulating capital. The measure of its success will be unprecedented compound annual revenue and net asset growth rates resulting from business unit expansion across a broad geography and range of human services.

INDUSTRY BACKGROUND

The behavioral health and social services industry (the "industry") is defined here to comprise the approximately 7,000 private nonprofit and for-profit companies that provide services in the following segments: behavioral health and substance abuse, developmental disabilities, juvenile justice, child welfare, and special and alternative education. These services are typically administered by state and local government agencies on behalf of children or others with limited capacity to voice their own needs or desires.

Federal and state governments have played a central role in shaping competition in the industry because they are both capable of licensing and regulating providers and among the largest buyers of services. With the growth of the welfare state in the 1960s, the delivery of industry services shifted largely from government to private nonprofit organizations. These nonprofit providers became increasingly reliant on fees paid by public agencies for survival because at the same time they were receiving fewer charitable contributions. Public policies have therefore been the key drivers of an industry historically characterized by low entry barriers, high exit barriers (specifically for nonprofits), few threats of substitute products or services (the noteworthy exception being pharmaceuticals), limited supplier bargaining power, and little rivalry among existing competitors.

In 2004, after two generations of rapidly growing revenues, the industry began a transition to maturity as segments such as developmental disabilities experienced (between 2004 and 2006) the slowest increase in state spending on community and institutional services per $1,000 of statewide personal income in the previous 30 years (Braddock et al., 2011). The impact of industry maturity on behavioral health and social services has been similar to that seen in other industries and has included: (a) more competition for share as revenue growth has slowed; (b) greater purchasing sophistication by (largely government) buyers; (c) competition focusing on greater cost emphasis; and (d) falling provider profits. Perhaps of greatest importance for the many small nonprofit providers in the highly fragmented industry, rapid growth can no longer be relied on to compensate for strategic errors, poor execution, or inadequate capital structures.

To date, the traditional response to industry maturity—consolidation—has been thwarted due to the large number of nonprofit service providers. Despite clear evidence for economies of scale and scope, nonprofit providers lack the capital or management capabilities required to execute roll-up strategies and yet continue to face imposing exit barriers.

As public funding mechanisms have shifted from cost-based and fee-for-service arrangements to managed-care and, more recently, to risk-sharing arrangements, the dominant position of nonprofit providers has been challenged by the emergence of both publicly traded and private for-profit providers. These for-profit market participants may have much greater financial and human resources than their nonprofit counterparts, which enables them to share financial risk with payers. While we have estimated that for-profits comprise only about 15% of industry providers, consolidation efforts undertaken by the industry's for-profit providers have led to the creation of four firms (National Mentor, Res-Care, Providence Service Corporation, and the behavioral health division of Universal Health Services) with revenues in excess of $1 billion. (The largest independent nonprofit human service providers have approximately $500 million in revenues.) This growth in for-profit providers has been accomplished despite their having been largely limited to transactions with other for-profit providers due to legal, regulatory, and judicial barriers facing for-profits that acquire nonprofits, including both overt and subtle public policies that favor nonprofit providers.

Still, there has been no response from the vastly larger nonprofit industry segment to this threat to nonprofit hegemony. Understanding why nonprofit providers have eschewed consolidation—and why that is about to change as the nonprofit business model evolves—requires knowledge of key differences between nonprofit and for-profit organizations and the ways in which these differences impact their business models and strategies.

A PRIMER ON NONPROFITS

Nonprofit organizations are a creation of state law, whereas tax exemption is primarily a function of federal tax law. Tax-exempt status confers two potentially significant benefits on nonprofit organizations: They pay no taxes with respect to net income on charitable activities, and donors may deduct contributions to most tax-exempt entities. To secure a nonprofit designation and tax-exempt status, nonprofit organizations agree to serve one or more specified public purposes and to accept a prohibition on the distribution of profits, which must instead be reinvested to further the organization's charitable purpose. Nonprofit organizations have no owners, and they are self-governing.

The absence of an ownership interest has at least two significant effects on the operation of nonprofit organizations: It limits access to capital because there are no equity investors, and it dilutes governance by impairing ownership's traditional role as a constraint on management's pursuit of private interests. The limited access to capital further hinders nonprofit providers' ability to invest in facilities, technology, management, and working capital. It also handicaps the capacity to finance participation in industry consolidation. As a result of these restrictions, nonprofit providers have grown almost exclusively through de novo development, and there are no national nonprofit consolidators. This evolution of the nonprofit sector has concurrently served the interests of nonprofit leaders, who have demonstrated a predictable reluctance to pursue the scale economies associated with business combinations at the risk of their own personal positions.

As a consequence, the nonprofit segment of the industry remains fragmented. A search of the Internal Resource Service (IRS) Form 990 tax returns for 2009 in the GuideStar database reveals approximately

1,900 nonprofit human service providers with revenues of $5 million or more. The distribution of these nonprofits by annual revenue is presented in Figure 2.1.

While these circumstances would seemingly pave the way for industry consolidation led by for-profit providers, this outcome has been thwarted by multiple obstacles. Foremost among these is the widespread belief among nonprofit trustees that the profit motive is incompatible with the mission of providing behavioral health and social services, compounded by the preference of many public officials and payers for nonprofit providers. In the absence of financial distress, these factors have often precluded nonprofit providers from responding to business combination proposals from for-profit consolidators, and there have been no nonprofit consolidators. Thus, nonprofit governance confronts a situation in which it has been unable to achieve scale in an industry that is entering maturity, yet it is unable to exit due to the self-imposed absence of a market for corporate control. The resulting excess capacity in the maturing industry suppresses the margin expectations of would-be consolidators, whether nonprofit or for-profit. This outcome is not serving the public interest, and recognition of this has initiated a variety of public policy responses.

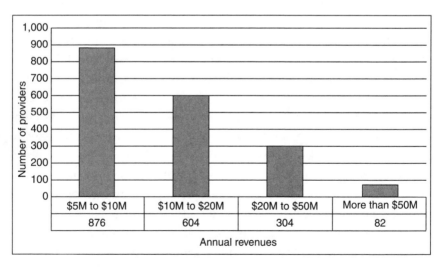

Annual revenues	$5M to $10M	$10M to $20M	$20M to $50M	More than $50M
	876	604	304	82

FIGURE 2.1 Nonprofit providers by revenues.
Source: GuideStar.org.

These responses have included the introduction of new forms of incorporation by various state governments. A low-profit limited liability company, or L3C, is a legal form of business entity that was created to bridge the gap between nonprofit and for-profit investing by providing a structure that facilitates investments in socially beneficial for-profit ventures. To date, L3C legislation has been adopted in nine states. Another alternative enacted in seven states is the "B corporation," which also combines elements of for-profit and nonprofit corporate forms. Other proposed innovations include social impact bonds. Each of these reactions is intended to address the capital access limitations inherent in the nonprofit corporation structure, ultimately enabling nonprofits to achieve critical mass while reducing unit service costs.

THE CHANGING INDUSTRY ENVIRONMENT

Changes in the industry as a direct result of legislation, including the 2010 Patient Protection and Affordable Care Act (ACA) and the 2008 Mental Health Parity Act, have been widely publicized but are hardly the only shifts impacting the industry. Hoping to gain lower costs and better value, the service delivery system is moving toward integrated behavioral health models that rely on evidence-based treatments augmented by technology and focused on outcomes. The traditional and expensive alternatives, particularly inpatient and other out-of-home treatment options billed by unit of service, are discouraged. Consequently, inpatient costs as a percentage of total behavioral health expenses have declined sharply, while substitute products such as pharmaceuticals, telehealth, and other technology-enabled forms of support continue to play a growing role in the service delivery system.

Such shifts in service delivery will have a significant impact on Medicaid, a major payer for industry services. On June 30, 2009, Medicaid enrollment stood at 46.9 million—approximately 15% of the U.S. population—and is expected to increase by 16 million participants following the full implementation of the ACA (Holahan, Clemans-Cope, Lawton, & Rousseau, 2011). Expected increases in states' Medicaid costs range from $21.1 billion to $43.2 billion over the years 2014 to 2019

(Holahan & Dorn, 2010). These increases in Medicaid enrollment and costs are occurring at a time when state revenues have remained 7% below prerecession levels as of the third quarter of 2011, and their fiscal challenges also include managing education and criminal justice systems. Collectively, these circumstances compel public officials to pursue opportunities aimed at reducing state expenses, in part by changing the way they contract for services and in part by privatizing some functions that were previously performed solely by government.

Shifts in financing arrangements prompted by new legislation and changes in service delivery have taken the form of risk-based contracting. These contractual arrangements require substantial capital capacity coupled with vastly improved accounting, information, and management systems, leaving most nonprofit organizations, which possess modest equity, at a distinct disadvantage. The capital shortfall cannot be simply addressed through the issuance of tax-exempt bonds, because tax-exempt financing is typically restricted to "bricks and mortar" investments. Thus, the shifts in financing encourage nonprofits to affiliate in order to create more robust balance sheets.

Pervasive capital constraints have had a decidedly corrosive impact on industry leadership. A 2006 study conducted by CompassPoint and the Meyer Foundation queried 2,000 nonprofit executives and found that three quarters of them did not plan on being in their present positions in 5 years (Bell, Moyers, & Wolfred, 2006). More recently, Challenger and Gray reported that health care and nonprofit organizations had the highest chief executive officer (CEO) turnover during the first quarter of 2012.

Collectively, market trends are compelling providers to evolve dramatically different care delivery systems, new management practices, and new strategies—in essence, an entirely new business model—in response to the paradigm shift.

PREVAILING NONPROFIT INDUSTRY BUSINESS MODELS

The industry's nonprofit business models have historically been program centric, differentiated primarily as a consequence of their sizes as measured by their annual revenues. As a result, providers typically transition from one generic business model (Osterwalder, 2007) to another in three stages, as summarized in Figure 2.2.

Development Stage:[a]	Stage 1	Stage 2	Stage 3	New Business Model
Geographic Market:	One Community	One Region or State	Multi-State	National

Market Segments:
  Customer Segments:
  Program Segments:
	
	One
	One
		
		One
		Several
			
			Two or More
			Multiple
				
				All
				Multiple

Value Proposition:	Activity/Unit of Service Unit Cost: Low Volume: Low Complexity: Low	Activity/Unit of Service Unit Cost: Moderate Volume: Low Complexity: Low	Activity/Unit of Service Unit Cost: Low and High Volume: High Complexity: High	Outcomes Unit Cost: Low and High Volume: High Complexity: High
Distribution Channels:	Public Agency Case Managers	Public Agency Case Managers/Public Managed Care Agencies	Multi-State Public, Private Managed Care Case Managers	Multi-State Public, Private Managed Care Case Managers and Direct to Consumers
Customer Relationships:	Local Public Payer/ Donors	Local and State Payer/ Donors	Local, Multi-State, Managed Care Payers, Federal Grants, Private Pay	Local, Multi-State Managed Care Payers, Federal Grants, Private Pay
Revenue Streams:	Few, Cost-Based, Revenues Highly Concentrated	Multiple, Constant Fee- Base, Some Diversification	Multiple, Constant Fee-Base, Substantial Diversfication	Outcome-Based Risk Sharing, Broad Diversfication
Key Resources:	Founder/Director	CEO? Other Human Resources	Capital/Management Team/Other Human Resources	Capital/Management Team/Tech./Brand/Other Human Resources
Key Activities:	De novo, Outpatient	De novo, Outpatient or Inpatient/Residential	De novo, Outpatient and Inpatient/Residential	Affiliations and Acquisitions
Partner Network:	Independent	Collaborative	Partnering	Acquisitive
Cost Structure:	Labor Intensive	Labor Intensive	Labor and Capital Intensive	Capital, Technology, and Labor Intensive

FIGURE 2.2   The nonprofit business model.

[a]For more regarding Development Stages, see Osterwalder, 2007.

The Stage 1 business model is typical of nonprofit human service providers with revenues of less than $10 million. These providers characteristically offer a single service within a single community (e.g., an outpatient behavioral health service or a residential service for developmentally disabled persons) that is funded by a single public payer, such as a county department of human services. Individuals or families receiving service might be referred by a public agency case manager, likely do not present with multiple chronic conditions, and can likely be served at low cost. These providers most often will have limited histories and capital, and fees are often earned under low-risk, cost-based contracts. Many Stage 1 providers are led by their founders, who often possess additional product-related expertise.

Stage 2 providers comprise those with revenues of $10 million to $50 million. These providers have evolved to offer a number of services (e.g., behavioral health and substance abuse outpatient services, or residential and vocational services for developmentally disabled persons) regionally or statewide, and they are funded by multiple public payers. Individuals or families receiving service might be referred by public agency case managers or managed care organizations, and some of these clients have service needs of moderate complexity, entailing moderate expense. These providers may have histories of 10 years or more but still lack significant capital due to revenues derived under a combination of cost- and fee-based contracts. Many providers transition to leadership by nonfounders in the course of Stage 2.

Stage 3 providers comprise the largest and best capitalized group. This structure offers a broad array of services for children, adults, and families in multiple states, and organizations may be funded by numerous public and private payers. Individuals or families receiving service might be referred by public agency case managers, Medicaid, or private managed-care organizations. These providers typically have long histories and have likely accumulated substantial capital, much of which is invested in real estate. Revenues are earned from many payers, and diversification of revenue streams has been a key driver of corporate strategy.

The typical Stage 1 organization structure consists of a single nonprofit tax-exempt enterprise that houses both service operations and fundraising, if the organization engages in any formal fundraising efforts. Stage 2 organizations frequently incorporate a separate charitable foundation to administer fundraising efforts and to separately house the net capital accumulated by the developmental efforts. Stage 3 providers usually adopt a holding company structure that includes multiple nonprofit providers, each a de novo venture established to address some unmet community need and each typically focused on a specific program. A venture may even operate in several different states. In these Stage 3 organizational structures, the parent company frequently operates as a management company in an effort to benefit from scale economies.

This evolution of organizational structures has little impact on capital accumulation but significant impact on nonprofit governance. The decision to create a foundation in Stage 2 adds significantly to the aggregate number of nonprofit enterprise trustees. Expanded board participation becomes unwieldy as Stage 2 operations become more complex, giving rise to trustee term limits during the stage when organizational founders are succeeded by professional managers. Trustee term limits tend to exacerbate the information asymmetry between nonprofit trustees and nonprofit management, increasing agency costs. The commercial world's antidote to agency costs—a market for corporate control—has not been operational in the human service industry historically, but the changing industry environment offers a catalyst. Payers increasingly demand integrated services that provide better outcomes at lower costs, and these demands are enforced through risk-sharing contracts that require larger, better-capitalized providers.

THE PREVAILING FOR-PROFIT BUSINESS MODEL

While the industry's for-profit consolidators include both publicly traded and private corporations, each pursues roll-up strategies supported by a similar business model. Roll-up strategies seek to create value in fragmented industries by combining a multitude of smaller organizations into one larger company. A skilled, experienced management team can create scale economies, and the consolidated enterprise will receive significantly higher valuation multiples than will those connected to the acquired entities individually. The key value drivers associated with this strategy are capital and exceptional management.

At the inception of a roll-up, investors—often private equity firms—fund a management team comprising industry experts who proceed to acquire a strong platform company. (Industry platforms typically have about $40 million in revenue and EBITDA [earnings before interest, taxes, depreciation, and amortization] of $5 million to $8 million.) Following the initial platform acquisition, a series of regional add-on transactions is pursued while a search commences for platforms in other regions of the nation, in order to expand both geographic coverage and product lines, and ultimately lead to a nationwide network. The relentless focus on growth via mergers and acquisitions typically leads roll-ups to enter multiple program and customer segments in an effort to maximize top-line revenue growth and scale economies. Customers include local and state agencies, managed care, and national insurers.

Revenue streams tend to be fee based and broadly diversified—the evolutions of ResCare, National Mentor, and Providence Service Corporation all followed this path.

Successful execution of a roll-up strategy promises substantial rewards stemming from the competitive advantages in the emerging marketplace that are associated with scale. Creation of a nationwide service network will enable large providers to enter into risk-sharing contracts that cover large numbers of beneficiaries over broad geographies at competitive prices. Concurrently, scale will facilitate accelerated rates of growth as the economic downturn compels smaller industry participants to exit. As the industry consolidates, the scale achieved by the consolidators will enable them to leverage the growing costs of technology and compliance over a large revenue base, and subsequently to erect barriers to entry. The marketplace will reward these developments with growing multiples.

With the economic downturn and disarray in capital markets since 2008, industry roll-ups have had to deal with a dearth of transactions in recent years. The pain experienced by the industry's leading for-profits has been mirrored by increasing financial distress at some of the industry's largest nonprofits. As the economy enters its sixth year of negligible economic growth, pressure grows on providers with weakening balance sheets to reassess strategic alternatives. With their structural, financial, and managerial advantages, for-profit roll-ups seem to be the likely beneficiaries, but national nonprofit consolidators, invigorated by new business models and refined strategies, might still emerge.

THE NEW NONPROFIT INDUSTRY BUSINESS MODEL

Ventures that transform industries require more than innovative ideas, careful planning, and a capable management team; timely market introduction is also critical. The current recession has resulted in an extended interval of constrained capital access for small companies, low-valuation multiples, and modest deal flow. In anticipation of the Fed's intent to maintain low interest rates for an extended interval, the likelihood of an increase in capital gains and income tax rates, and the growing pressure on government to curtail budget deficits, the timing is ideal for industry consolidation.

Capitalizing on the opportunities presented by the new human service paradigm will require nonprofit providers to adopt a new business model that is both capable of pursuing traditional consolidation strategies and supported by innovative organizational and financial designs. The goals of the new business model will be twofold: rapid growth supported by improved governance and new mechanisms for accumulating capital. The measure of success will be unprecedented compound annual revenue and net asset growth resulting from business unit expansion across a broad geography and range of human services.

Strategic Characteristics

The new nonprofit business model must support a strategy that recognizes managing mergers and acquisitions (or *affiliations*, as change-of-control transactions involving two or more nonprofits are termed) as an organizational skill that can serve as a key element of differentiation. Actions stemming from this awareness include:

- *Adopting management-designed and board-approved formal acquisition criteria that encompass a defined acquisition process with an emphasis on speed of execution*

  Speed of execution is critical because a successful nonprofit consolidator must overcome the presumption that nonprofits are incapable of executing expedient transactions. Expedience is also important because the present economic environment is at a peak for nonprofit consolidators due to the unprecedented levels of interest rates, the large number of nonprofits facing leadership transitions, and pervasive concerns about a long-term decline in public funding for industry services.

- *Utilizing both experienced, in-house business development professional(s) and business brokers to maximize deal flow because nonprofit transactions frequently entail an extended sales process*

  The extended sales cycle associated with nonprofits results from the absence of any ownership interests to drive transactions, cumbersome trustee processes, and a lack of top management sophistication. Because these roadblocks cannot be overcome through the actions of the nonprofit consolidator, it is necessary to generate robust deal flow via a business development organization that is able to create, pursue, and monitor that flow.

- *Recruiting legal counsel who is knowledgeable and experienced in both mergers and acquisitions and nonprofit law, along with outsourced due diligence support (at least for the initial transactions)*

Legal counsel plays an important role in the execution of commercial transactions, and this role is critical in nonprofit transactions because of the many unique aspects of nonprofit affiliations. The nonprofit consolidator's counsel will routinely be placed in the position of not only drafting the affiliation agreements and the numerous resolutions to be adopted by the boards of the consolidator and the target nonprofit, but also educating the target's general counsel on the nuances of the pertinent law. Transactions may also involve additional complexities associated with outstanding tax-exempt debt.

The acquirer's due diligence process seeks to both minimize risk and create future value. These important dual objectives should be entrusted to experienced experts, and any attempt to maintain this capacity in-house risks delayed execution for consolidators pursuing multiple transactions simultaneously but having only limited control over the pace of these transactions. This circumstance invites the outsourcing of due diligence, given the historically low volume of industry affiliations and a shortage of industry-experienced experts.

- *Willingness and capacity to deploy capital to induce nonprofit targets with superior growth prospects to affiliate, specifically targeting nonprofit organizations that are facing transitions in the executive suite*

Given that transactions with distressed providers—a historical mainstay of nonprofit affiliations—do not augment capital capacity by definition, these should not have a role in a consolidation strategy. To facilitate transactions with healthy nonprofits, cash transfers from the consolidator to the new affiliate on the closing date will become a fundamental ingredient of nonprofit affiliation strategy. These cash transfers are useful to nonprofit consolidators because they do not constitute a "price," they shorten the sales cycle, and they enable consolidators to more rapidly increase net assets.

Organizational Characteristics

Implicit in its strategic focus on consolidation, the new nonprofit business model will incorporate a holding company organizational structure to facilitate changes in corporate control, capital formation, efficiency, transaction processing, and risk mitigation. Specifically, the holding company organization structure can be expected to yield the following benefits:

- *Entry into new geographic and program markets quickly and at scale.* The nonprofit holding company structure enables a nonprofit consolidator to easily add multiple affiliates via a change in the affiliate's articles of incorporation. These articles are typically amended on the closing date to provide that the parent company (or an existing affiliate of the parent company) will become the sole member of the new affiliate, with the power to appoint and remove affiliate trustees among other things.
- *Avoiding relicensing and contract assignments.* Growth by affiliation or acquisition—that is, deals analogous to stock transactions rather than asset purchases—enables the parent company to avoid relicensing existing services and assigning the affiliate's various contracts and receivables.
- *Acquisitions in addition to affiliations.* The nonprofit holding company structure facilitates a nonprofit consolidator's acquisition of for-profit as well as nonprofit providers. In many circumstances, the acquired entities will continue to operate on a for-profit basis, blurring the distinction between nonprofit and for-profit providers.
- *Centralized governance.* The sole-member organizing principle allows for centralized control and decision making at the parent-company level, including centralized decision making with respect to capital allocation. These are essential tools for executing strategies involving goals related to care integration,

technology investment, achieving scale economies, and management accountability.

- *Enhanced management performance.* Execution of a successful growth strategy focused on acquisitions requires engaging senior executives with skills and experience that vary from those of traditional nonprofit leaders and incentivizing them with contractual arrangements that better align organizational and management interests.

Financial and Operating Characteristics

Implicit in its strategic focus on consolidation, the new nonprofit business model will incorporate an intense focus on capital accumulation and scalable information systems because these are fundamental requirements for executing consolidation strategies. Financial and operating policy implications of the new nonprofit business model include the following:

- *Balance sheet focus.* The financial management of industry nonprofits has historically focused on the income statement, with boards typically adopting annual budgets for revenues and expenses with scant attention (if any at all) to pro forma balance sheets. In the new nonprofit model, financial goals are measured by referring to changes in net assets because capital capacity is a function of net assets and optimum size is driven by capital capacity.
- *Defining and targeting optimum organization size.* The optimum size of a nonprofit organization is the maximum level of revenue that can be prudently sustained given the available capital and the nonprofit's expectations of future market conditions. The purpose of nonprofit budgeting is to quantify operating and business development activities that are intended to achieve optimum size over time.
- *Value creation through affiliations.* Nonprofit business combinations can be expected to create increases in net assets each year that are equivalent to multiples of annual operating profits during the industry's consolidation phase, with first movers likely reaping the greatest benefits. Nonprofit affiliations differ from commercial

acquisitions in that there is typically no purchase price, although there will frequently be a cash transfer from the parent to the new affiliate at closing. (There is no accounting impact at the enterprise level stemming from these cash transfers because the consolidated financial statements of the parent include the cash of all affiliates. In short, cash transfers, in contrast to the purchase price in a commercial transaction, amount to merely moving cash from one pocket to another.) Importantly, the assets, liabilities, and net assets of new affiliates are consolidated in the financial statements of the parent company effective on the closing date at their fair market values. Therefore, virtually every affiliation increases the parent's net assets at closing. Essentially, the first affiliation begins a positive cycle in which every deal creates value for the parent, and this incremental value can enable each subsequent transaction as long as there is sufficient cash available to pay any required cash transfers.

- *New focus for the CEO.* With business combinations having by far the greatest impact on growing net assets, nonprofit CEOs must make planning, business development, and board relations top priorities, leaving operations and fundraising to other executives. In so doing, the nonprofit CEO will be essentially mirroring his or her for-profit counterparts.

IMPLICATIONS AND SPECULATIONS

The adoption of the new nonprofit business model will have significant implications for the industry. Most obvious will be increased efficiency resulting from better allocation of the capital available to the industry. Less obvious, but equally significant, the new business model will improve governance, management, and systems, leading to increased competitiveness and, ideally, effectiveness.

Because a small cadre of regional and national providers generates a growing proportion of industry revenues, it seems likely that distinctions between service providers related to their tax statuses will diminish. With the evolution of regional and national brands, it seems probable that the best-capitalized and best-known nonprofits—often faith-based organizations—will be the last nonprofits standing.

I expect that they will prove to be formidable foes to even the largest industry competitors once greater industry concentration creates increased regulation and cements lobbying as a distinct competence in the industry.

BEST-PRACTICE SHARING: A LOOK AT THE CHANGING NONPROFIT HUMAN SERVICE AND SOCIAL SECTOR INDUSTRY AND ITS PRIVATE-SECTOR COMPETITION

Arianne Sellers

With the implementation of the Patient Protection and Affordable Care Act, human service organizations will see an increase in Medicaid participants and a push toward diverse, impact-based initiatives through technological advancement and collaboration. Structurally, for-profit companies have the upper hand. They have the flexibility to invest in and reduce the cost of services while nonprofits continue to focus on their missions—losing sight of the operative goals of efficiency and solvency. For-profits have also smartly used their corporate clout to gain political influence, by both using the dollar-driven political process and engaging officials through lobbying to ensure access to contract bidding and policy issues such as unfettered reimbursements for government services such as Medicare.

The trend toward human service corporatization may seem inevitable, but it is not. Innovative solutions for engaging the competition exist and are already producing sustainable growth in the nonprofit arena. These sound concepts not only hold the key to nonprofit survival but also create greater impact by addressing society's growing needs. Consolidation strategies in the nonprofit human service sector through acquisitions, affiliations, and mergers, among other business model changes, are imperatives going forward for strengthening the sector's stability and renewing its political presence. By remaining flexible as organizational networks with a clear focus on the future market, nonprofits are primed to utilize the recent disruptive forces for inspired growth.

The salient point in the comparison of for-profit versus nonprofit human service entities often emerges as a question of quality. Previous public service privatization ventures, such as child welfare systems, have historically done little to boost service quality or innovation. In this era, can large corporate interests be expected to serve societal needs over the demands of shareholders while also promising affordable solutions to seemingly insurmountable welfare concerns? Many of the publicly traded for-profit human service organizations specifically list criticism of privatization and operational quality as a risk their investors must consider. Ultimately, are the limited American tax dollars distributed through government agencies for these services to varying degrees producing a good return on our investment? Perhaps, when it is equipped with the proper tools for adaptation and business savvy, the nonprofit sector can remain a more dominant force in the human service industry, setting the standard of excellence for all players. The study of a number of for-profit examples will illustrate the current trends and impacts in addition to the actual and potential consequences. While I provide no definitive road map to a market revolution, I do intend to highlight the many complexities nonprofits face in America as they seek a competitive edge.

The Human Service Industry

The human service industry umbrella encompasses a range of social and behavioral health services, such as disability programs, youth development, mental health and crisis intervention, and employment, housing, and child and family services. Before the 1960s, these efforts were considered largely governmental. But through welfare state growth, it became common for nonprofit organizations to serve communities through public agency funding, such as Medicaid, with legislative efforts focused on fostering these partnerships. Approximately 7,000 private for-profit and nonprofit companies exist in the market today (Fee, 2013, p. 1).

Demand for community services has increased owing to economic hardship, but the current political climate and tax revenues ensure only basic funding. Nonprofit organizations rely more heavily on government financing than do for-profits, and they also tend to have a donor base that can be similarly impacted by economic conditions. Societal needs continue to rise and nonprofit organizations are spread thin, while competition for additional funding through foundations, mergers, and acquisitions has become quite common, both with other nonprofit networks and increasingly with for-profits as well. Fortunately, nonprofits are somewhat shielded from for-profit acquisition because of existing transaction regulations, such as legal boundaries; that has not, however, mitigated corporate expansion. Even traditional political motives in nonprofit preference may not be safe for much longer.

Service Finances

The human service industry contains an estimated 15% for-profit competitors, both private and publicly traded. Smart consolidation strategies include bolstering existing financial and human resources by establishing a wide variety of social and behavioral health services through a single firm, the largest of which all post revenues of more than $1 billion. Some for-profits have also creatively sidestepped state regulations that mandate solely nonprofit government contracts by actually integrating nonprofits into their business models through service delivery and management services (Fee, 2013, p. 2). As a result, large portions of that billion-dollar revenue (and in some cases, all of it) can be traced directly back to the federal and state government coffers. Shareholders of publicly traded human service companies are advised that this dependency can be an investment risk because so much income is tied to agency funding in the form of extensive contracts for services and reimbursement for care.

This vital government arrangement increases the need for close legislative tracking and political organizing by for-profits to maintain their current payout structures and also to potentially gain access to more opportunities for privatization under new legislative agendas. These large for-profit firms can, and do, donate thousands of dollars to political entities such as state and local parties. They contribute directly or through structures such as political action committees (PACs) and super PACs to influence electoral and government policy outcomes. Large corporate contributions of "soft money" have increased dramatically in the past decade (Center for Political Accountability, 2012). The IRS permits this fundraising through several tax-exempt classifications, including 501(c)(4) social welfare organizations, which function as partnerships to support shared policy and political interests, like those in the human service industry (Internal Revenue Service, 2014). In the for-profit sector, these entities have become more popular than PACs because they are purportedly "advancing broad community interests" and are therefore not subject to scrutiny by the Federal Election Commission, while they are still shielded from the critique of shareholders and consumers (McIntire & Confessore, 2012, p. A01). A *New York Times* review reported that in 2011, corporate donations to these social welfare groups not only increased but also were specifically intended to impact and guide public policy at all levels of government (McIntire & Luo, 2012, p. A01). By contrast, nonprofits, as 501(c)(3) tax-exempt organizations, cannot participate in any partisan electoral activities and are limited to some lobbying efforts only in the form of organized advocacy.

Mission Failure and Rebirth

At the heart of the nonprofit sector's lack of competitive edge in the human service industry lies a fundamental difference in operational philosophy. The publicly held and private for-profit structures are Wall-Street-responsive entities with bottom-line concerns that constantly aim to reduce operational costs to ensure maximum revenue. Tom McLaughlin, a nonprofit consultant and author, describes the mission-based nonprofit business considerations of corporate structure as detached from the nonprofit identity. This includes the various "trappings of corporate structure" and any common administrative instruments such as software or management processes. He states: "People do not feel positively about an organization because they have a fondness for its corporate structure" (McLaughlin, 2010, p. 14). While the nonprofit human service sector has evolved through several stages, including the 1990s' growth in mental health programs, many experts like McLaughlin agree that the industry is again ripe for restructuring. It is apparent that the for-profit sector has the economic strength to continue experimenting with and innovating ways to corner the market. However, through similar business structures and political influence, these developments can inspire the new nonprofit design as well.

First and foremost, the trends of network building and business consolidation strategies (e.g., mergers, acquisitions) within the nonprofit community must be expedited in order to facilitate the larger adaptation strategies. Common concerns are always based in maintaining the missions and reputations of individual nonprofit organizations. With the alliance of competing or redundant services, networks can return to their goals through the shared delivery of high-quality human services and measurable impact (Alliance for Children and Families & Baker Tilly, 2011, p. 11). Furthermore, this cooperative system will simplify mobilization strategies for legislative advocacy and political influence. With shared resource databases of known donors and advocates for the various human service nonprofit entities, the sector can enable more grassroots organizing and citizen lobbying of government officials within the traditional 501(c)(3) tax-exempt model. The creation of 501(c)(4) social welfare agencies in the nonprofit arena is growing in popularity, and these can be quite useful because they allow for more flexibility in political influence and policy making with the added benefit of primarily anonymous donation policies. Established social welfare initiatives can then also be financially supported by outside organizations that share the same policy-shaping goals, such as labor unions.

The next nonprofit sector evolution must include careful consideration of operational procedures and financial models, with innovative integration of market-responsive strategies. In the human service industry, there is a growing government preference for multiyear contracts, often in the form of risk-based contracting. This requires not only healthy financials but also streamlined processing of support services such as accounting and management. Because such an arrangement requires significant capital, it is again pertinent for nonprofits to seek consolidation strategies within the sector to help combine funding sources and reduce competition among those with the same mission-based services. Some industry analysts also recommend that nonprofits integrate a for-profit subsidiary into their business structures to help ensure fiscal solvency (Fee, 2013, p. 5). Even within networks of providers with no formal business relationships, partnerships among diverse service providers should be encouraged to help reciprocate the shared goals of high-quality, impactful social and behavioral health services. Technology advancements in all aspects of the human service business model can be expected to push nonprofit adaptation and expenditures as well, while also fostering innovation in program delivery.

In addition, maintaining localized influence and public integration will be a priority within the nonprofit sector. This creates a sense of ownership among the residents, supporters, and community members who utilize the human services, leading to donations, advocacy support, and legislative engagement. Although for-profit acquisition strategies often include the expansion of regional service delivery by way of calculated local market introductions and subsequent expansion, nonprofit entities can rely on the organically altruistic sentiment generated by their organization structures.

One example of political and financial prowess in the nonprofit world is AARP (formerly the American Association of Retired Persons). While AARP is not in the human service industry, many of their successful strategies reflect the recommended changes for nonprofits in all sectors, such as the diversified business structure beyond the charitable organization itself. The AARP model specifically contains a 501(c)(4) arm for lobbying and a for-profit corporation that licenses the organization's brand name for use by other business entities. Impressively, this nonprofit group was actually the third most prolific lobbying organization in 2008 and continues to grow in membership and strength (Carney & Capital Research Center Staff, 2010, p. 2). Despite its lack of direct human service involvement, AARP has held significant policy-making power on the same issues that impact the human service industry, such as health care reform.

CONCLUSION

While we may study the many strategies by which the nonprofit sector of the human service industry can sharpen its competitive edge, perhaps the most critical fact in this examination is that the number of Americans who require social and behavioral health services is growing; in some areas, this need is increasing at a staggering rate. Every individual who receives quality care, whether it be in the form of an HIV screening or a free tutoring program for a mentally disabled child, is one step closer to contributing to our society in a positive way. Humans are, after all, social creatures who value community collaboration in caring for one another, and nonprofits exemplify this very mission. Government tax dollars may be in short supply, but human services programs should not be the first on the budget chopping block; nor should the neediest people in our society be further denigrated by programs operated from Wall Street rather than being grounded in social impact performance measurements. Prepared with adaptive tools, the nonprofit world will continue to identify the future needs of our citizens and to develop solutions while for-profits will be reviewing the financial risk involved.

REFERENCES

Alliance for Children and Families & Baker Tilly. (2011). *Disruptive forces: Driving a human services revolution.* Milwaukee, WI: Alliance for Children and Families. Retrieved from www.alliance1.org/disruptive-forces/executive-summary

Bell, J., Moyers, R., & Wolfred, T. (2006). *Daring to lead 2006: A national study of nonprofit executive leadership.* San Jose, CA: CompassPoint Nonprofit Services and the Meyer Foundation. Retrieved from www.compasspoint.org/sites/default/files/docs/research/194_daringtolead06final.pdf

Braddock, D., Hemp, R., Rizzolo, M. C., Haffer, L., Tanis, E. S., & Wu, J. (2011). *The state of the states in developmental disabilities 2011* (The Arc National Convention Edition). Boulder, CO: Department of Psychiatry and Coleman Institute for Cognitive Disabilities, University of Colorado. Retrieved from www.stateofthestates.org/documents/SOS%20FINAL%20REVISED%20EDITION2011.pdf

Carney, T. P., & Capital Research Center Staff. (2010). *AARP: Retired people never had it so good.* Washington, DC: Capital Research Center. Retrieved from www.capitalresearch.org/2010/04/aarp-retired-people-never-had-it-so-good

Center for Political Accountability. (2012). *A primer on corporate political spending.* Washington, DC: Author. Retrieved from www.political accountability.net/index.php?ht=d/sp/i/6346/pid/6346

Fee, K. (2013). The emerging market for nonprofit control: Business model implications. *Philadelphia Social Innovations Journal,* January

2013. Retrieved from http://www.philasocialinnovations.org/site/index.php?option=com_content&id=507%3Athe-emerging-market-for-nonprofit-control-business-model-implications&Itemid=31

Holahan, J., Clemans-Cope, L., Lawton, E., & Rousseau, D. (2011). *Medicaid spending growth over the last decade.* Kaiser Commission on Medicaid and the Uninsured. Washington, DC: The Henry J. Kaiser Family Foundation. Retrieved from www.kaiserfamilyfoundation.files.wordpress.com/2013/01/8152.pdf

Holahan, J. & Dorn, S. (2010). *What is the impact of the Patient Protection and Affordable Care Act (PPACA) on the states?* (Timely Analysis of Immediate Health Policy Issues, June 2010). Washington, DC: Urban Institute and Robert Wood Johnson Foundation. Retrieved from www.urban.org/UploadedPDF/412117-impact-patient-protection.pdf

Internal Revenue Service. (2014). *Common tax law restrictions on activities of exempt organizations.* Washington, DC. Retrieved from www.irs.gov/Charities-%26-Non-Profits/Common-Tax-Law-Restrictions-on-Activities-of-Exempt-Organizations

Kania, J., & Kramer, M. (2011). Collective impact. *Stanford Social Innovation Review, 9*(1), 36–41. Retrieved from www.ssireview.org/articles/entry/collective_impact

McIntire, M., & Confessore, N. (2012, July 1). Tax-exempt groups shield political gifts of businesses. *The New York Times,* p. A01.

McIntire, M., & Luo, M. (2012, January 6). After Santorum Left Senate, familiar hands reached out. *The New York Times,* p. A01.

McLaughlin, T. (2010, August 1). Who are you? *The NonProfit Times, 24*(13), p. 14. Retrieved from www.thefreelibrary.com/Who+are+you%3F+mergers+don't+mean+lost+identity.-a0239359110

Nonprofit Finance Fund. (2011). *2011 state of the sector survey.* New York, NY. Retrieved from www.nonprofitfinancefund.org/files/docs/2011/2011survey_brochure.pdf

Osterwalder, A. (2007). *How to describe and improve your business model to compete better.* Melbourne: La Trobe University. Retrieved from www.setoolbelt.org/resources/830

3

Identifying the Right Partnership Strategy

Thomas A. McLaughlin

EDITORS' OVERVIEW

Following on Chapter 2's discussion of how the nonprofit sector can take advantage of for-profit collaboration strategies to expand its reach and impact, noted partnership expert Tom McLaughlin discusses how to choose the type of partnership that will be most effective for your organization.

CREATING PARTNERSHIPS: STRUCTURING AND MANAGING ARE VALUABLE TOOLS

Partnership is a word that comes up frequently today in nonprofit management conversations, and for good reason. Challenging economic conditions, declining funding, and demographic realities are combining to renew the nonprofit sector's support of joint action.

These kinds of actions can take many forms. But unlike many words rooted in law and business, the term partnership still has a soothing ring and seems to offer the promise of a new way of doing things.

Perhaps, the most interesting aspect of a partnership is that the term is rarely used in a legally and financially correct way. In its most precise incarnation, a partnership is simply a formal relationship between two or more individuals or business entities that is intended to help the partners accomplish one or more mutually desired goals. Subject to a few requirements of the Internal Revenue Service (IRS) and perhaps local governments, a partnership is considered formed simply by the acceptance of a partnership agreement.

Because the concept of a partnership is so flexible, these kinds of technical requirements do not matter much for our purposes. There is a spirit to the term, not just the letter, that makes a successful partnership of just about any kind.

Clear Goals

The essence of a good partnership is that it should help each partner achieve specific goals. For this reason, each partner needs to be clear about the goals it is trying to achieve. Ideally, this level of corporate goal should be related to a strategic objective.

By definition, a partnership should help each partner achieve something that it could not achieve on its own, or could not achieve as well.

This principle highlights the rather mundane nature of a partnership. It is primarily a vehicle for accomplishing objectives. There is a tendency to romanticize the use of partnerships, but in the end, they should be primarily a tool.

ECONOMIC PARTNERSHIPS

It helps to think of partnerships as having two dimensions: the purpose and the level of integration necessary to make the partnership work. Figure 3.1 shows the four primary types of partnerships: corporate, operations (programs), responsibility distribution (administrative), and economic. The "easier" partnerships start at the bottom, and each horizontal level represents the level of integration that

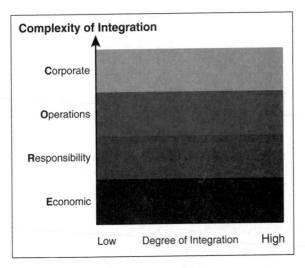

FIGURE 3.1 The four primary types of partnerships (corporate, operations or programs, responsibility or administrative, and economic) and the degree and complexity of integration required for each.

is necessary, from low on the left to high on the right. For this purpose, let us concentrate on the lower three levels. A partnership that involves legally integrating two or more corporations is considered a merger, but for our purposes, we are primarily focusing on nonmerger partnerships.

Partnerships with economic goals are usually the easiest to form because they have a limited focus. If a nonprofit with an unneeded building gets together with another nonprofit that simply needs more space, the partnership is nicely delineated on the far left side. In practice, this is the kind of commercial transaction that takes place every day. But if the same partnership involves, say, a major renovation by the nonowning corporation, the demands of the partnership become more complicated. The parties would move horizontally to the right on the economics continuum because they would need to integrate their economic choices more tightly. If two nonprofits decide to form a partnership to jointly acquire a building, they would move their partnership to the far right.

ADMINISTRATIVE PARTNERSHIPS

There is a great deal of interest in administrative partnerships. These can range from partnerships that concentrate on a single backroom service to those that involve colocation. The nonprofit center movement is a good example of highly integrated administrative partnerships. These kinds of partnerships are harder to carry out than simple economically oriented ones because they involve complex recurring procedures that touch on sensitive areas of any nonprofit's operations.

In many ways this model is a way to "outsource" certain functions, except to a group in the same building, not in a different country.

Administrative partnerships thrive on two elements: scale and standardization. Most administrative functions—such as payroll services, accounting, and information technology (IT)—are composed of many small transactions repeated in high volume over and over. This kind of scale is fertile ground for reducing costs, but only if the transactions occur in compatible formats in predictable ways. For a detailed treatment of this topic, see "It All Adds Up" in the January 2011 issue of *The NonProfit Times*.

It is the need to bundle large numbers of transactions within a single system that pushes administrative partnerships to the right, toward higher integration. Major corporations and large universities first caught onto this model in the last century when they began forming in-house service centers. This seems to have been the origin of the term "shared services," which has come to define just about any administrative combination.

Notice that inherent in the shared services model is a certain concession to scale and standardization. To get greater scale one may need to assemble many nonprofits, and getting standardization means giving up some basic operational choices. But when the reward is lower costs, the trade-off may be highly desirable.

PROGRAMMATIC PARTNERSHIPS

Partnerships forged around program services are the pinnacle of contractual partnerships that do not require corporate change. They are the most complex, and involve the most sensitive area of a nonprofit short of its corporate identity. They are also arguably the most difficult to organize and manage.

Partnerships at this level are difficult because of a phenomenon we think of as "pride of program." Most nonprofits take tremendous and justifiable pride in the services they offer, and that alone makes programmatic collaboration an unappealing option for many. Programs and services are so fundamental to an organization's mission that leaders of a group will fiercely protect them, making it difficult for one group to "expose" its programs to the possible inadequacies of another organization.

Brand protectiveness is at the heart of these reactions, as it should be. A good brand is an asset in every sense of the word, worth well more than the fundraising dollars it can bring in. Brand protectiveness is an organizational equivalent to the survival instinct in human beings. For this and other reasons, programmatic partnerships usually have one or more characteristics.

One common feature is what is known as *vertical integration*. This means that organizations at different but contiguous steps in a process will collaborate more readily than will those at the same step. For example, in an eastern gateway city, a medically oriented organization teamed up with a social service entity to greet incoming immigrants from all over the world. The partnership worked well because the medical and social needs of the new arrivals were met in a sensible fashion and because each group was skilled at handing off an individual or family to the other.

Program partnerships can also work well in time-limited or emergency situations such as natural disasters. The immediacy of the moment and the intensely shared mission can help overcome the natural we-do-it-better impulse. Of course, logistical snags and system breakdowns, common in these same situations, can hobble these temporary partnerships.

All of these tendencies combine to keep program partnerships toward the left, the less integrated area. It is "safer" there, with less risk to brand equity and more flexibility. There are many tacit partnerships in large communities and service systems. Organizations in an unofficial continuum of care typically develop institutional preferences for one or more different organizations to whom they refer consumers for the next step in the care process. The health care world has formalized many of these by creating large multicorporate systems, but the same organizational impulse can be seen in education, economic development, and community action programming as well.

Partnerships are a valid response to current trends. There are no partnership registries except in the case of actual legal partnerships. The handshakes or tacit agreements to the left side of the horizontal levels cannot be tracked but seem to be an always popular tool. Knowing how to structure and manage partnerships will be a valuable skill for the street-smart nonprofit manager in the future.

BACKROOM COLLABORATION: THE SECRET SAUCE OF WORKING TOGETHER REALLY IS NOT COVERT

Near the top of the category of "things that ought to work a lot better than they actually do" are backroom collaborations. There has always been a consistent level of interest in backroom collaborations among funders and many nonprofit managers, and the recent economic troubles have only accelerated it.

With its implicit promise of painless savings (except for the jobless employees in the backrooms), the concept is simple and appealing. It is also a lot harder to accomplish than most people expect.

Success in nonprofit collaboration around administrative functions lies in making the proper matches in the first place and then managing everyone's expectations. The most fundamental expectation to manage is the dreams of massive savings to be squeezed from a backroom collaboration. First, consider the mathematics of administrative collaboration. Assuming that the collaborating organizations are already spending in the range of 15% of total revenue, even a near heroic 10% savings in administrative costs will amount to less than 2% more to be spent on programming. Most organizations would be happy to have an additional 2% flexibility in their costs, but an administrative collaboration can be an awful lot of work to go through to get it.

This raises one of the hidden costs of backroom collaborations, which we call alliances. The staff time required to make them happen is almost always "extra" time, over and above the normal demands of day-to-day operations. This means that collaboration time is often a lower priority, squeezed out in favor of more pressing business.

Moreover, even in well-staffed partner organizations, it is often not clear how important the alliance is in the eyes of the senior leadership. This can be a recipe for frustration, which is why setting expectations properly is so important.

The Three Ingredients

All of these concerns can usually be managed by having clear-eyed expectations for what the alliance can reasonably be expected to produce, what it will take to produce those results, and how important the results are to the participants.

However, there are three essential ingredients in the secret sauce of backroom collaboration that are inherent in the participants' characteristics and that go beyond process considerations: standardization, replicability, and scale.

These are must-haves—without them, a backroom alliance is highly unlikely to succeed. Let us take each in turn.

Standardization

During the era of Henry Ford, it was said that customers could have a Model T in any color they desired as long as it was black. This quip gets at the heart of the economic proposition behind money-saving administrative alliances. Significant cost savings are rooted in standardized procedures.

On the face of it, administrative alliances would seem to be natural candidates for standardized processes. After all, money is money, right?

Well, not exactly. For one thing, money-handling procedures are not nearly as uniform as they appear to be. Just the fact that collaborating organizations use different software packages for the same purposes greatly increases the degree of difficulty in collaborations. And there are judgment calls about things such as officially recognizing revenue that can vary considerably.

Beyond the question of basic standardization is the effect of consumer preferences on administrative details. United Way facilities around the country discovered this many years ago when they worked on building a collaborative pledge-processing infrastructure. The simple act of accepting a pledge from a participating employer's workers took on significant administrative complexity. Lockboxes (post office boxes where contributions were sent) sometimes had to have a regional flavor and even recognizable local zip codes. The fear was that employees giving to workplace campaigns would be turned off by the Anywhere, U.S.A., message that local donors do not matter.

Pledge forms needed to be customized for each local United Way. Sometimes, different forms needed to be used for varied audiences. It would have been easier if everyone had been satisfied with black, but that is not the way of the 21st century.

The reason many nonprofit backroom operations are not standardized is that they tend to be put together in support of programs and services that are not standardized; each has different terms to refer to essentially the same thing. But even if a crosswalk between terms and services exists, no one can say for sure that the organizations are dealing with the same thing in the same ways.

Replicability

For administrative alliances to be successful, they must include replicable components. Closely related to standardization, replicability means not only that a process is based on standardized components but also that those components are regularly combined in the same way.

Human resource management is a good example of nonreplicable procedures. Because most nonprofits with fewer than 75 to 100 employees find it difficult to hire and retain a true HR professional, the smaller systems tend to have been cobbled together in a hodgepodge fashion. Combining the two systems into a single operation would yield few replicable procedures without a major overhaul of at least one but probably both.

The appropriately person-centered nature of so many nonprofits' services, though often a source of satisfaction to consumers and staff alike, works against replicability in a fundamental way. Without an overarching agreement about the service models using the administrative services, it is unlikely that two or more backrooms will have enough in common to maintain replicable processes.

Scale

Finally, for administrative alliances to be successful, the services being integrated need to have a certain level of scale, or size of operations. This requirement is grounded in basic economics. Low volumes of transactions will not support the added administrative effort needed to make an alliance work, and they may not even be sufficient to improve the quality of the work being done. In turn, this suggests that each participating organization has to be of sufficient size to support a minimum volume of activity and enough professional staff to match.

The corollary to this idea of a minimum number of participants is that it is very unlikely that small nonprofits (say, less than $3 million in revenue) will have the capacity to plan and execute their role in an administrative alliance. They probably do not have enough staff time, and there may not be a sufficient level of management capacity, either. This "administrative alliance tax" is the reason small organizations may be better off colocating rather than trying to build administrative alliances.

A strategic side note is worth mentioning here. There is a tendency today to think of administrative collaboration as a novel, nonprofit-centric idea. Yet there is a long history of for-profit entities' picking off a single function around which to build a kind of alliance.

For example, in the health care field, for-profit professional billing services have effectively created a narrowly focused "alliance" around a single package of billing software. The only reason these companies exist is that they captured the market before nonprofits thought of doing the same thing among themselves. Organizations in the newer and fast-growing parts of the nonprofit sector might have the chance to build their own version of such a company as an alliance—if they move quickly.

Administrative collaboration among nonprofits is worth trying. But the proper ingredients have to be in place. Any special sauce worth the money has to be standardized, replicable, and produced in large-enough quantities to satisfy all consumers.

COMMUNITY COLLABORATION FUNDS DEFINE CRITICAL JUNCTURE FINANCING

When the board and management of a for-profit company decide that it is time for a merger, they can easily learn about the applicable laws and regulations and the pool of advisers available to them. If they begin the process, they expect to pay for any related services out of current earnings or, in some cases, from future proceeds. When the board and management of a nonprofit decide that it is time for a merger or an alliance, they are on their own.

This imbalance of resources is especially harsh because nonprofits do not typically have extra earnings or future vehicles to tap for the inevitable additional costs of a serious collaborative effort. This is why local collaboration funds for nonprofits are beginning to sprout all around the country.

These funds, which rarely have similar names, may not even be designed similarly, but all share the same goal of making it easier to facilitate collaborations among nonprofits. With the lingering effects of the recession and the plentiful state and city budget crises, it is safe to assume that the demand for such assistance is only going to increase in the coming years.

What is less well understood, but ultimately perhaps more important, is that funding for collaborations is only the most immediate aspect of what is needed. The other missing aspect is an infrastructure robust enough to support collaborating organizations in ways other than financing. That infrastructure should consist of widely proven practices, experienced advisers, and well-tested laws and regulatory policies. Financing local collaborations is a way to jump-start that process, too.

Financing collaborations is not a new idea. The concept was written about in *The NonProfit Times, Exempt*'s sister publication, as far back as 1999. (See "Critical Juncture Financing," *The NonProfit Times*, December 1999.) At that time, it was noted that critical juncture financing "would be any kind of financial resource provided by a third party…to facilitate the successful transition of two or more nonprofit organizations to the next stage of their development." This remains a durable definition, and today, the evolution of nonprofit collaboration allows for building even further on that foundation.

COLLABORATE TO FUND

A good starting point for the community financing of collaborations is for the funders to model the behavior themselves. While this is not essential, if two or more funders can agree to pool resources, it sends a powerful message that collaboration is good for everyone. Funder collaboration also offers two other important benefits: the funding pool will be larger, and the administrative costs can be lower. Engaging multiple funders can lengthen the pool development time, of course, but the benefits should outweigh the costs.

Matching Funding With the Stage

Collaborations typically go through three distinct stages. The first is feasibility determination, in which the partners analyze their respective operations in the context of a possible mutually beneficial collaboration. The second is implementation planning, when the willing parties create a work plan for the collaboration. And the third is integration, the much longer stage when the newly linked organizations work out the day-to-day details of their relationship.

Collaborating nonprofits tend to prefer grants during the first or second stages of their work together. Collaboration activity is normally seen as discretionary because most available funds are put to everyday essentials, and also, collaboration tends to be seen as a new or one-time-only event, although this will probably be less true in the future.

In the integration stage, the commitment has been made and acted on and the organizations are planning a joint future, so there may be more of an appetite for loans and program-related investments, especially because capital may be needed for property acquisition or different information technology systems.

Grants also make more sense in the beginning stages because the organizations typically are not comfortable enough to risk their own capital on the process. This parallels another logical tendency of collaborating organizations. Because formal collaborations, especially mergers, are so new to most organizations, they are more willing to entrust the work to outsiders.

As the parties develop trust and the process grows more and more operations oriented, the nature of the tasks grows so similar to what the organizations are already doing every day that the participants often feel more comfortable doing those tasks in-house.

THE LOCAL INFRASTRUCTURE

Once the funding is in place and the fund has been designed, some funds might wish to simply process the applications. But the stronger argument is that community collaboration funds have a responsibility to help build ongoing local capacity for restructuring activities. There are many ways to do this, and here are a few of the stronger ones.

Record the Basics

Simply recording the basic information in a consistent manner will help a community. What types of organizations apply for the funding (use companies' National Taxonomy of Exempt Entities [NTEE] codes to look up the organization type)? For what purpose will it be used? At what stage are they when they apply? In a short time, these simple data will likely show significant trends that could be useful in the participating funders' other work.

Require a Success Metric

Collaborations should be carried out primarily to strengthen programming. This objective often gets obscured by those experienced in mergers of publicly held companies, who assume that nonprofit collaborations should produce cost savings. What they should produce is a community benefit, and because that benefit will be different in different situations, the important metric of collaboration will be whatever the participants settle on.

Record the Metric

Most mergers take several years to become operational. By requiring a success metric (or metrics) and recording it as part of the funding process, community collaboration funders can begin to build a record of which collaboration approaches work and which do not.

Know the Local Adviser Base

There are many different types of nonprofit advisers in every community, but until recently, few had any experience in nonprofit collaborations. Many of today's collaboration advisers were yesterday's strategy and development consultants, and their experience is still thin. A community collaboration fund can have a lasting impact just in the way it defines collaboration-related services.

Share the Knowledge

Community collaboration funds, singly and collectively, will produce valuable information about what works, what does not, and why. This is a good resource for local nonprofits and their funders and policy makers as well as for academics.

CREATE THE FUND

In concept, a community collaboration fund is simple to set up and administer. One or more organizations sets aside a designated pool of funds, solicits applications, and distributes the money. Three things are likely to surprise funders interested in such a vehicle.

First, the administration can be time-consuming. This is partly because the fund is a start-up operation and partly because many of a funder's normal files and tools either will not apply or will need to be modified for the collaborative approach.

Second, the fund must be marketed. This may seem counterintuitive, but even "free" resources need to be marketed. Further, the fund could need to "sell" the idea of collaboration before being able to sell itself. These are not difficult steps, but they can be time-consuming.

The trickiest difficulty is both cultural and administrative. Community collaboration funds, especially multiparty efforts, are not a common approach for most funders. Even more difficult, these funds attempt to build capacity among grantees in lieu of funding programs and services. While building capacity has been more popular among funders in recent years, the two inherent differences can be formidable barriers to execution.

Community-based collaboration funding is one of the most promising ways of strengthening programs and services. The nonprofit sector does not need to build the intricate patchwork of laws, regulations, and advisers that characterize for-profit mergers, but the sector does need support systems that help collaborating nonprofits avoid wasting their time in re-creating the wheel. Providing local capital for local collaborative solutions accomplishes all of these goals.

THE SUBSIDIARY: CERTAIN WORDS CAN BE VERY SPECIFIC

There are certain words that seem to practically cry out their message. One of those words is the term *subsidiary* as it is used to describe a particular kind of corporate structure. Here the word subsidiary seems to embody a subordinate position.

The phrase "take-over" is sometimes associated with the concept of a subsidiary. This offers a kind of double condemnation. In a freedom-loving culture, being a subsidiary of any kind reeks of lost privilege and status. But hold on: The story is more complicated than it seems. As the word is used here, subsidiary means a corporation that holds a certain position and is in a defined relationship with at least one other corporation. Some of that relationship is legally defined and even legally required. But a lot of it is left to the judgment of the corporations and their respective managers. This is why digging into the actual terms and requirements of subsidiary relationships may produce some surprising, counterintuitive results.

Accountability Versus Power

Although it might seem otherwise, the subsidiary structure is more about accountability and protection than it is about power. In a corporate sense, power often refers to the ability of a person such as a chief executive officer (CEO) or a department head to compel certain behavior on the part of those who report to that person. This is the classic power imbalance that is usually muted but that unmistakably underlies classic relationships in a corporation: The boss is in charge.

In a parent–subsidiary model, the word *parent* refers to the corporate entity that is in charge of the subsidiaries. It might also be called a holding company or a management company. There is a power imbalance between the two entities, but it is nothing like that between boss and employee. In fact, for those employed in a subsidiary, it is not unusual for the parent company to seem more as if it is located somewhere else on a cloud (and not the computer kind). The parent is a recognizable organization, but employees of each corporation may well regard one another as though they are simply citizens of moderately allied countries.

The reason for this apparent estrangement is that it is a by-product of a major advantage of subsidiaries: They represent boundaries. This is one of the most compelling reasons for them—corporate boundaries serve as a kind of firewall between the parent corporation and outsiders who might be intent on suing a subsidiary. Rarely does an aggrieved outside party succeed in attacking the parent company by first trying to go through a subsidiary. Lawyers refer to this as piercing the corporate veil, and it is rarely accomplished because each corporation is expected to stand on its own in all legal proceedings.

This is not a corporate version of dodgeball. Different types of services have different risk patterns, and there can be dramatically negative economic consequences for treating all services in a parent-subsidiary environment alike. For example, major hospitals that coexist in a complicated multicorporate structure will virtually always run nursing homes or home care services as subsidiaries. This is because a successful lawsuit against a hospital can potentially bankrupt a nursing home if it is part of the same subsidiary.

Boards of directors represent a good example of subsidiary corporations' roles in ensuring accountability. Not only will a smart parent company taking on a new subsidiary be open to the latter's board continuing, they might insist on it. Apart from the fact that the parent company board may need to take a crash course in running the new subsidiary, dismissing the board would destroy all institutional knowledge at the governance level.

Brand Management

Well-run nonprofits know how to manage their brand(s). While it is possible to manage a brand through many different departments—even through many different corporations—it is much easier if that brand has implicit boundaries. Brand management is a top-down function, which is why parent companies will not usually meddle in the promotion of a successful subsidiary's brand.

The Top Line, Not the Bottom Line

Many nonprofit board members and some executives feel that a successful merger should save money. This is a worthy goal, but subsidiary corporations still need CEOs, audits, executive staff, and other expenses. Skeptics will ask why a nonprofit should do something like this if it does not save money.

The answer is that while the bottom line is important, in many sectors of the nonprofit field today, the top line—revenue—is even more important. Hospitals began creating numerous parent–subsidiary models two and even three decades ago. Arts groups are doing a similar version of the same thing in many locations.

Behavioral health care providers in many states are entering a new phase of consolidations that often involve parent–subsidiary models. Providers of services to develop mentally disabled persons in some states are facing similar changes.

Integrated systems of care almost always have more power with funders who themselves are often enlarging their scopes as well than do individual organizations; larger arts groups can reach bigger audiences, etc. When parent–subsidiary models are used in these situations, savings may or may not be realized, but what often does happen is that the newly enlarged organizations, simply put, increase their power at the bargaining table.

This kind of scaling up is fairly rare in the nonprofit world, which is why subsidiary corporations are still rarely found outside of hospitals, universities, research institutions, and other large entities. But forces such as managed care, shifting risk management requirements, and health care reform are providing fertile ground for more parent–subsidiary relationships.

WHAT YOU SHOULD DO

What should you expect if your current organization becomes a subsidiary of a larger one? Or, if you are a CEO contemplating making your organization a subsidiary, what should you attempt to achieve in the process? The key indicators are much the same for both viewpoints.

Board Integration

The parent company's board will likely become the sole corporate member of the new subsidiary, giving it official control of the entity. This creates a legal tie in lieu of a "purchase," which for-profit corporations routinely carry out. In practical terms, however, this too is an accountability mechanism, not a control technique.

In practice, wise parent companies will seek board integration. Ideally, the subsidiary board of directors will contribute at least one or two members to the parent company board. This is important symbolically, and it also helps build cultural compatibility. Note that these individuals must abruptly do double duty between the board of origin and the new parent board, but it is nearly inconceivable to create a smooth integration of parent and subsidiary any other way.

How to Treat the Brand Name

In most cases, this element will be an early topic of negotiations, and it may be especially important for the smaller organization. Brand name philosophy—and the systems that support it—should be an early topic of discussion unless the future subsidiary has a damaged brand or the parent has a far stronger one.

The CEO's Role in the New Entity

For obvious reasons, this is both a symbolic and a very real indicator. While most of a subsidiary's employees are unlikely to have intense, sustained contact with the parent company, the CEO should be deeply involved in these relations. Ideally, the subsidiary CEO's role will be articulated and important.

Shared-Funder Positioning

Another key indicator is the new subsidiary's role in future relationships with a shared funder. The parent company is likely to take the lead in these negotiations, so the most important cue will be how the subsidiary CEO's role changes. Note that this and the previous indicator are the only instances in which the staff of the parent and the subsidiary play the classic boss–subordinate roles.

Money Decisions

Relatively small, ordinary financial decisions may be largely unchanged by a subsidiary designation. But acquiring and using capital for things such as buildings or specialized equipment are almost certain to change in some fashion. The decision-making process around major expenditures will often change, and some decisions will be made, or at least affirmed, at a higher level than before.

SUBSIDIARY PREROGATIVES

There is a whole category of what we would call subsidiary prerogatives that could change—or remain untouched. These are things such as purchasing decisions, marketing, fundraising and development activities, and personnel management practices. The future direction of these kinds of items is a good potential clue about future relations between the two entities.

Subsidiary corporations are a valid and effective way of managing risks, distinguishing brands and other assets, and approaching consumers in different yet coordinated ways. Most nonprofits will not become part of a parent–subsidiary structure, but external demands and internal strategies are boosting the use of this time-tested option.

HOW SHOULD WE GET TOGETHER? THERE REALLY ARE NOT THAT MANY CHOICES IN MERGERS

As nonprofits consider working together ever more closely in response to economic conditions, or just from a realization that collaboration makes sense, there are constant questions about how to make it work. Often at the heart of these questions lies a fundamental choice about the collaboration model that the participating organizations either do not recognize or are confused about.

For many, the situation grows murkier when they take up questions that cannot be answered until they answer the fundamental one: Exactly how should we get together?

In our venti, half-soy, nonfat, organic, iced, double-shot, gingerbread frappuccino world, it may be surprising to hear that the choices for exactly how two or more nonprofits should actually get together come down to two: contractual or corporate restructuring. There are variations and shades aplenty, of course, but at the highest level, the choice is binary.

THE IMPLICATIONS

Here is what the two choices mean. The term *contractual* is used as a loose descriptive term for collaborations between two entities whose joint objectives require some kind of ongoing operating documentation. It may be an actual contract with enforceable provisions, contingencies, and so on, or it can simply be a written agreement.

In some cases, there may not be a written agreement between the principals but rather a shared commitment to take parallel action. The collaboration can be designed to be limited in scope or to expire after a certain period, or in a few rare cases, it can be designed to continue indefinitely.

By contrast, a corporate collaboration changes in some ways the corporate identities of both participating organizations. The possible variations and subtleties are limitless here, but the essence of the change is that both corporate "vehicles" experience some form of change as a direct result of the collaboration.

Clearly, there are major differences between these two choices. An obvious one is that change at the corporate level is almost certain to be longer lasting. A less obvious difference is that there will likely be many additional changes throughout both organizations as well, at the program level, for example, as well as at the board and staff levels. A nonintuitive corollary is that change at the corporate level is likely to lead less rapidly to changes at other levels, if only because the new organization has more time to implement the changes. A contractual collaboration, on the other hand, might lose value and momentum if it does not result in speedy reforms. For example, if two or more entities create a contractually based joint purchasing program, they are likely to lose interest if it does not produce savings within just a few months.

How can two or more organizations decide which type of collaboration to use? A combination of their objectives in entering into the collaboration, as well as the facts of the situation, usually makes the decision straightforward. The chart in Figure 3.2 illustrates some common collaborative objectives along with the type of collaboration that will be most likely to accomplish organizations' joint goals. The intention of the chart is to suggest the most likely type of connection that two or more nonprofits will use to accomplish a specific goal. The two right columns suggest the most likely choice of collaboration structure for those desiring to accomplish a single specific goal. For situations involving multiple goals, the decision will probably entail weighing

Goal	Corporate	Contractual
Achieve financial stability	✓	
Acquire or manage real estate	✓	
Capture administrative savings	✓	✓
Carry out a joint venture		✓
Create or enhance a brand	✓	
Fill a leadership vacancy	✓	
Improve governance	✓	
Increase administrative effectiveness	✓	
Increase fundraising	✓	
Manage risk through insurance	✓	
Offer joint programming		✓
Reposition organizations in market	✓	
Rework programming	✓	
Save money	✓	✓

FIGURE 3.2 Comparison of corporate versus contractual partnership goals.

the overall portrait that emerges and making a decision based on where the majority of the goals fall. Note that a corporate structure change will typically involve two or perhaps three organizations trying to accomplish a series of goals whereas a series of contractual goals could well involve many different contractual partners.

In some cases, the goals have been listed as being achievable through either choice, but that does not mean that the choices are equal. For instance, capturing administrative savings can be done through either contractual or corporate means, but a higher level of long-term administrative savings is usually only achievable through a corporate change. Administrative effectiveness is listed as achievable via corporate change because this is more of a qualitative goal, in contrast to saving money, which can be accomplished in many different ways.

Goals with a corporate focus, not surprisingly, should only be attempted via corporate change. Acquiring real estate through a partnership (a contractual vehicle) as opposed to a single corporation can certainly be done, but it is often messy and raises tricky questions about fairness and risk and reward sharing. Brand management is best done with a corporate focus, as is fundraising—these things reside at the heart of organizational identity. Joint programming is always possible, but wholesale rethinking and repositioning of programs is virtually impossible to carry out without a single point of responsibility such as that found in corporations. Again, see Figure 3.2.

In collaborations as in architecture, form should follow function. Collaborating nonprofits will find that their joint efforts will flow more smoothly if they start out being clear about their ultimate goals.

ON THE DOTTED LINE: IN PRAISE OF MANAGEMENT CONTRACTS

The newly hired executive director seemed promising at first. He was the first full-time person in that position and had a year, more or less, of similar experience; it seemed like a good fit.

There was a small fire in one of the residential programs. No one was hurt. It was clearly a resident's fault (smoking), but it scared everyone, and left a mess from the sprinkler system. After a few months, it became clear that the founding board members—the board president and two of her closest friends and neighbors—could not let the incident go. And then one of the program managers began to distance herself from the new executive and the rest of the staff. Rumor had it that she was disappointed at not being considered for the executive director's job. In a small organization, the dysfunction was potent.

The founding board members began to talk among themselves, and then the founder began to make stronger and more persistent inquiries of the executive director about "how things are going." The inquiries became hints, and the hints culminated in a "we have to talk" conversation. Within months, the executive director left to take a different job in a different town.

Variations on this scenario happen all the time. Some readers may even recognize it from personal experience. The board members would eventually have begun to say that they had made a hiring mistake. The former executive director would have attributed it to inexperience and a convergence of odd events and unfortunate misunderstandings.

An impartial observer might say: "These things happen all the time. Who cares?" And this would be correct—these things do happen all the time. A more thoughtful observer, however, might note that executive directors and the small nonprofits that hire them might need to make mistakes like these because it is all part of the parties' learning and development.

But what if the organization had been in a situation in which it needed stability in the executive's chair and the newly hired executive director had suddenly bolted for greener pastures? What if the organization had been accused unfairly of some kind of malfeasance and needed the skills and experience of its executive director to clear its name, yet the person took advantage of the moment to go to a larger competitor?

These are all problems of executive absence from the other side. People will identify more with an individual CEO's need for stability, yet nonprofits need stability in the executive chair for their own purposes. Stability in the CEO chair is valuable.

MANAGEMENT CONTRACTS

One answer to this two-party problem is a simple yet surprisingly underutilized one: management contracts. At its simplest, a management contract is a binding document signed by the organization and the executive that outlines the relationship between the two. Management contracts often have unique provisions and varying purposes. For the moment, concentrate on their use solely from the perspective of how best to ensure that executives remain in place for a specified period of time. Nonprofit World is a trusting sector, but there are still situations in which board members may want a legally acceptable contract to ensure the services of the CEO (and other executives) for a period of time. Here is a spotlight on a few.

Founder Transitions

Particularly appropriate in view of the number of nonprofit founders and CEOs who are at or near retirement age, management contracts can be a good way to ensure the continuity of a successful nonprofit. This should happen in the context of an organization-wide planning effort to move through the CEO transition as smoothly as possible. Ideally, the contract will incorporate a succession plan. These can be particularly smooth when the CEO takes the initiative to map out the timeline and the steps that would be needed for a glitch-free handover.

Holding onto Gold

Boards that are particularly satisfied with their CEOs may want to consider management contracts because of the value inherent in an effective leader. There is a tacitly competitive CEO marketplace in metropolitan areas with large numbers of similar organizations. The competitiveness often causes individual CEOs to rule out ever working for the competition, but this does not happen all the time. When a defection occurs, it can be damaging organizationally and culturally.

Mergers

Nonprofit mergers are prime situations for management contracts. It is often very difficult to get two organizations with sitting CEOs to consider a merger because each fears losing his or her job. This is a myth, because there are ways of having two CEOs (or comparable positions) in the same organization, although verbal reassurance is not as powerful as a contractual obligation.

Here is another combination scenario in which to consider management contracts for each CEO. Suppose a CEO plans to work for a small number of additional years and wants to use that time for a smooth transition. The partner is headed by a CEO who is acceptable to the other entity as a replacement for when the CEO retires. Each CEO gets a management contract with his or her current organization, but the succeeding CEO's contract is at least a year or two longer than the retiring CEO's. As long as the two CEOs can create a working relationship, this scenario would work well. And, as in the above note, neither individual necessarily needs to lose the CEO title as long as the structure is put together correctly.

Succession From Within

If the plan is to eventually replace a retiring CEO with an internal candidate, board members may want to have parallel and complementary contracts with each executive.

Litigious Environment

Although it does not happen often, some nonprofits operate in a litigious environment. Social welfare organizations—501(c)(4)s—are more likely to be in this situation, but it can also happen to public charities under unusual circumstances. CEOs in this kind of situation may be well advised to have a management contract that spells out in detail any provisions for legal assistance provided by the organization.

THE 3 Ps

What goes into a management contract? The easy answer is whatever the organization and the CEO want to include. There are some norms—think of them as the 3 Ps: pay, power, and perks. Management contracts are valid legal instruments that are best structured by lawyers, but the 3 Ps will always touch on the majority of the concerns.

Some typical provisions include payment for the length of the contract except if the person is terminated for cause. Power provisions are harder to build in for obvious reasons. The essence is that executives will not lose the power in their positions except as a result of the most egregious of behaviors. The terms and conditions should be very clear and, ideally, should probably be the product of a mutual discussion, and contract renegotiation should be built in to account for unusual circumstances.

Are you worried about rogue board members, intrusive regulators or donors, or an inexplicable burst of bad public relations? In this ethical and self-aware sector, these things do not happen very often, but remember the executive director described above? No nonprofit executive is immune. Maybe it is time to break out the legal pen.

NOTE

Portions of this chapter were published in the following volumes of *The NonProfit Times*:

"Backroom Collaboration," Vol. 24, No. 1, January 15, 2010

"How Should We Get Together? There Really Are Not That Many Choices in Mergers," Vol. 26, No. 3, March 1, 2012

"Creating Partnerships: Structuring and Managing Are Valuable Tools," Vol. 27, No. 3, March 1, 2013

"The Subsidiary: Certain Words Can Be Very Specific," Vol. 27, No. 15, November 1, 2013

"On the Bottom Line: In Praise of Management Contracts," Vol. 28, No. 2, February 1, 2014

A separate portion was originally published in *Exempt* magazine, a sister journal to *The NonProfit Times*: "Community Collaboration Funds Define Critical Juncture Financing," October/November 2011.

4

Building a Culture of Collaboration

*Ashley Del Bianco, Kate Rivera, Judith Bernstein-Baker,
Natasha Keleman, Ashley Tobin, Gretchen Shanfeld,
and Annette Mattei*

EDITORS' OVERVIEW

As noted in previous chapters, strategic partnerships can take many forms: affiliations, collaborations, full mergers, and others. This chapter and the next look at how some successful nonprofit agencies began building a new culture of partnership within the nonprofit sector through successful collaborations, less formal arrangements under which all involved parties maintain their independent governance but work together for a common cause.

THE FREEDOM RINGS PARTNERSHIP: COMMUNITY-FOCUSED COLLABORATION

Ashley Del Bianco and Kate Rivera

The Freedom Rings Partnership was formed in 2010 to tackle the problem of the digital divide in Philadelphia, where many of the residents lack reliable Internet access. The partnership seeks to address this problem by increasing access both at computer labs and at home and by providing computer training that is integrated into broader social services programs. By taking a collaborative, community-based approach, the partnership has seen success in connecting residents to resources that allow them to improve their quality of life as well as in fostering capacity building and best-practice sharing in local nonprofit organizations.

The Digital Divide in Philadelphia

Think about all of the things you use the Internet for in your daily life. Now imagine not having that access while most of the people around you do. That is the plight of an estimated 41% to 55% of Philadelphians who do not have Internet access at home. This lack of access—and the related resource and information gap—is termed "the digital divide."

Basic computer proficiency and Internet access are necessary for finding a job; attaining an education; connecting with family, friends, and the broader community; and accessing information about health, benefits, and transportation. Lack of Internet access correlates strongly with individuals who have lower incomes, those with lower education levels, and minorities such as African Americans and Hispanics.

The Freedom Rings Partnership

The Freedom Rings Partnership was formed in 2010 to take a cross-sector, collaborative, and focused approach to improving computer literacy and Internet access for the most disenfranchised and low-income Philadelphia residents. The partnership received two federal grants totaling $18 million under the Broadband Technology Opportunities Program, a part of the federal stimulus funding. Leveraged with matching support, this represented an infusion of $27 million focused on a community-based approach to the problem of digital inequity in Philadelphia.

Our goal is for all Philadelphians to have access to the Internet and know how to use a computer. We accomplish this by providing Internet access through our free public computer labs, called KEYSPOTs; promoting low-cost, in-home Internet options; providing training on computer and Internet use; and creating a broad-based awareness campaign about the benefits of computer and Internet access. This approach combats the main barriers to Internet access: price and lack of perceived relevance.

We help people like Kathy, who enrolled in a jobs program and took KEYSPOT computer classes at one of our partner organizations, People's Emergency Center. As a single mother, Kathy's goals were to develop basic computer skills, "find a decent job," and buy a computer so she could help her daughter with her schoolwork. She completed basic computer training, began a specialist certification, and secured employment.

So far, the partnership has

- Launched more than 80 KEYSPOTs, or public computer centers, throughout Philadelphia
- Provided more than 170,000 hours of computer training to more than 17,000 participants
- Served more than 266,000 clients with free computer access
- Reached more than 4.1 million people with broadband adoption awareness impressions through an extensive branding and marketing campaign

Led by the City of Philadelphia's Office of Innovation and Technology and the Urban Affairs Coalition, the partnership comprises more than 50 organizations, including Drexel University, the Philadelphia Parks and Recreation Department, People's Emergency Center, Philadelphia FIGHT, Media Mobilizing Project, the Free Library of Philadelphia, Philadelphia OIC, One Day at a Time, and Youth Outreach Adolescent Community Awareness Program (YOACAP). KEYSPOTs, our public computer and training locations, are located primarily in existing community-based organizations (the ones named above in addition to other social service organizations) in neighborhoods with low broadband adoption. Computer use and training are integrated into the organizations' other programs to provide a more comprehensive social services approach. Rather than approaching computer training as being about the technology, our focus is on the needs of our clients and how technology can support their goals.

While the federal funding necessitates a somewhat hierarchical structure, the partnership is highly collaborative, with working groups that make decisions and share best practices in training, marketing, website development, technology management, and evaluation. This practice has fostered remarkably close bonds between partnership organizations, encouraging the sharing of information and referrals among organizations.

Early Highlights From Research and Practice

By codeveloping impactful partnerships with community-based organizations, higher-education institutions, municipal government, and residents themselves, the KEYSPOTs are beginning to demonstrate positive effects on individual and neighborhood social outcomes. They serve as hubs for computer and Internet access but also as safe, pleasant community spaces where goal-driven, learner-centered education happens. Although each center is geared toward the interests of the particular populations it serves, the partnership unites around the belief that forming and strengthening relationships through purposeful learning is central to engaging citizens and building community.

The partnership has engaged the New America Foundation's Open Technology Institute to conduct an independent evaluation of the program's outcomes and the effectiveness of the partnership's strategies for improving digital access and adoption in Philadelphia. Additionally, researchers from Rutgers University's School of Communication and Information are conducting a qualitative analysis of the tangible social and economic effects of broadband adoption in Philadelphia's low-income communities. While the data collection is ongoing and the analysis is preliminary, formative evidence from both studies indicates that the partnership's community-based approach is having a positive impact on digital access and digital literacy outcomes in Philadelphia.

The emerging research themes illustrate the benefits of a community-embedded strategy for doing this work. Initial research from Rutgers University suggests that successful digital training programs are embedded within existing community organizations, specifically those that provide other services, for example, health care, education programs, housing services, or workforce development. With the integration of technology tools and expertise into existing organizations that already work with Philadelphians in their neighborhoods, residents are engaging in learning, work, and community life in new and extended ways. For example, the early evaluation analysis indicated that KEYSPOT participants were developing their technology skills not only to search for employment and develop their resumes but also to gain new skills to apply in the workforce. While programs may offer direct access to employment, participants cite access to new social networks and material components such as a quiet place to work as being equally important to their experience. The social bonds that participants are forming at KEYSPOTs are contributing to stronger community connections; participants are volunteering at the KEYSPOTs, creating media to share, and using their skills to communicate with the wider community.

By providing technology training that is relevant to participants' goals and needs, we are integrating digital learning into the organizational missions of our diverse network of partners. One partner has decided to expand its adult literacy programming because participants who initially came for technology training have asked for further learning opportunities. The organization is recruiting both adult learners and tutors among KEYSPOT participants and the immediate community. Another partner now hosts two technology labs and has been able to expand its youth arts programs with extensive media production opportunities. A third partner has built new and highly popular programs for women in particular immigrant communities to learn both English language and technology skills.

The partner organizations are also strengthening relationships with one another by sharing promising practices and participating in partnership-wide professional development activities. The partnership has codesigned, sponsored, and led two training roundtables for all of the KEYSPOT lab assistants and trainers; at these sessions, peers shared practical advice, instructional methods, and content resources to enrich the knowledge base of the KEYSPOT community. Partners have also established both formal and informal networks for referring participants for additional digital literacy training and for other social services in which particular partners have expertise, such as housing, recovery services, and educational programs.

Ultimately, the success of the Freedom Rings Partnership rests with its ability to reach and consistently serve the diverse communities and individuals of Philadelphia. Philadelphia is a major city with a large population with significant social needs and few community resources, and the geography of the digital divide is starkly apparent. The Freedom Rings Partnership purposefully selected locations so that the neighborhoods that were least likely to have broadband access would be served. To assess this measure of effectiveness, the partnership and its evaluators developed a workstation user survey, a brief, anonymous, and voluntary questionnaire that appears at initial log in at every KEYSPOT terminal. The survey collects basic demographic information from participants who are 18 years of age or older. The analysis of survey results to date indicates that KEYSPOTs primarily serve African Americans, women, and people older than 55 years, as well as Hispanics, of whom the majority are women. These promising results strengthen the partnership's commitment to sustaining the community-based, mission-driven strategies that are reaching and serving communities with new access to critical technology and enhancing residents' abilities to participate in society as workers, learners, and citizens.

Looking to the Future

The Freedom Rings Partnership has demonstrated the tremendous success that a focused, collaborative, and community-based approach can have on a significant citywide problem. As the federal grant funds wound down in 2013, we continued working to ensure that we would be able to sustain and grow these collaborations. As our experience and research show, community involvement and support have been crucial components of our success.

POLICY CHANGE TO AID IMMIGRANT YOUTH SPURS COLLABORATION: THE FORMATION OF THE PHILADELPHIA DEFERRED ACTION NETWORK

Judith Bernstein-Baker and Natasha Keleman

The Movement Toward a Dream

On June 15, 2012, President Obama announced a significant shift in immigration policy: Under a new program referred to as Deferred Action for Childhood Arrivals, or DACA, his administration would protect certain young undocumented immigrants from deportation and issue them work permits and Social Security cards. Nationally, an estimated 1.4 million youth were eligible to apply for DACA at the time. The youth targeted under this program are American in every sense of the word except for their immigration status. Many were brought to the United States as infants and had completed high school or were attending college here. They were valedictorians and babysitters, musicians and meat packers, law students and restaurant workers. Without stable immigration status, these youth were relegated to working in the underground economy. They faced uncertainty about their futures, knowing that at any time they could be forcibly returned to their countries of birth—countries with which they probably had few ties and where they possibly did not speak the language. Without legal work authorization, these young immigrants worked in marginal jobs and were often subject to exploitation.

DACA is not a permanent solution for these young immigrants, but rather a stopgap measure implemented by the president after the Development, Relief, and Education for Alien Minors Act, better known as the DREAM Act, languished in Congress. President Obama's DACA policy does not go as far as the DREAM Act would have, and eligibility is limited. Unlike the DREAM Act, DACA does not provide a pathway to citizenship for childhood arrivals, and it does not enable beneficiaries to obtain any public benefits or student grants or loans. To be eligible, applicants must have lived in the United States for 5 years, have entered before 16 years of age, and have been at least 15 years old and below 31 years old as of June 15, 2012. But under DACA, those who meet these conditions are allowed to work legally and are protected from deportation for a renewable period of 2 years.

DACA Creates a Need

Immediately after the June 2012 announcement of DACA, nonprofit immigration service providers, advocates, and community-based groups began receiving calls requesting information and assistance. Eligible DACA applicants had to weigh considerable risks and over-come significant challenges to apply. With thousands of youth in the Philadelphia region eligible to apply for DACA, no single immigrant legal service provider or advocacy organization had the capacity to meet the need for outreach and legal assistance.

Judith Bernstein-Baker, executive director, and Philippe Weisz, man-aging attorney, of HIAS Pennsylvania (the Hebrew Immigrant Aid Society) felt that their organization was well positioned to convene a net-work of local immigration advocates and service providers to address DACA. The Immigrant Youth Advocacy Project of HIAS Pennsylvania specializes in legal assistance to unaccompanied, abused, and neglected immigrant youth and has strong relationships with stakeholders. Weisz convened a meeting of advocates and service providers to prepare a coordinated response. The Welcoming Center for New Pennsylvanians provided space for the first meeting and led the group in developing a preliminary fact sheet to dispel myths and explain what was known about the program at the time. A week later, the group met with repre-sentatives of the Philadelphia Foundation, the Samuel S. Fels Fund, and Philanthropy Network Greater Philadelphia to alert them to the oppor-tunities and needs created by DACA. Foundation staff encouraged the organizations to continue their collaboration and to hire one coordina-tor who would do extensive outreach to set up community information sessions, recruit pro bono attorneys and other volunteers, and leverage each group's resources.

Putting Young People First: The Collaborative Model

The groups joined together to form the Philadelphia Deferred Action Network (P-DAN) to conduct outreach to eligible immigrant youth, provide screenings and legal assistance, recruit and mobilize pro bono attorneys, and ensure swift processing of applications; each group brought resources and skills to the table. HIAS Pennsylvania agreed to act as fiscal sponsor and to write grant proposals. The Pennsylvania Immigration and Citizenship Coalition (PICC) was selected as the coordinator host site, given its advocacy mission and structure as a coalition organization. PICC hired a "DREAMer" whose own DACA application had been approved to coordinate the effort; the network's leadership team felt strongly that a young immigrant who had been involved in advocacy was the best person to identify outreach strategies. The Welcoming Center drafted the first informational flyer, leveraged media coverage, and offered its extensive mailing list for outreach purposes. DreamActivist Pennsylvania reached out to its network to inform its members about DACA. The Interpretation and Translation Department of the Nationalities Service Center (NSC) translated the information sheets into 10 languages. Juntos and the New Sanctuary Movement agreed to conduct outreach and organize community meetings. Ceiba spread the word among its contacts in the Latino community. Immigration legal service providers NSC, Esperanza Immigration Legal Services, Catholic Social Services, and HIAS Pennsylvania began staffing community clinics and providing free or low-cost legal assistance to individuals along with a private attorney, David Bennion, a trusted counselor to immigrant youth activists.

It quickly became clear that P-DAN had the capacity to meet the need for legal services in Philadelphia but that surrounding counties and rural areas were struggling. P-DAN therefore shifted its focus to organizing legal clinics in areas that lacked low-cost immigration legal services. Attorneys from P-DAN member agencies and pro bono attorneys volunteered to staff the clinics outside of Philadelphia. P-DAN utilized a number of models of service delivery to enroll as many young people as possible. In one model, community members attended an information session to learn about the DACA requirements and determine if they were eligible. If they were deemed eligible, they received a follow-up individual appointment to meet with an immigration attorney. In another model, community members came to an information-and-screening session and, if they were deemed eligible for DACA, were asked to return two or three weeks later with documents for a pro se clinic where their application was reviewed by a nonprofit representative or a trained pro bono attorney. Volunteers helped at these group clinics by copying documents, caring for children, and providing interpretation.

P-DAN also leveraged the skills of Harvey Finkle and Mark Lyons, a local photographer and storyteller, respectively, to develop a short video featuring stories and photos describing the lives of five local DACA applicants. This video was used by the entire collaborative to educate the public about DACA and put a human face on the young immigrants who sought to end their marginalization. "Even though DACA is a partial fix, it provides a way young people can come out of the shadows and begin to see a future; it enables us to see what contributions they can make to our region," noted Philippe Weisz.

P-DAN was a successful collaborative model that utilized members' strengths and encouraged coordination and cooperation instead of duplication and competition. Member organizations were quick to come together to develop a coordinated response to the new policy and to secure funding from multiple sources to support outreach and legal services. Each member organization recognized the value of the other partners. The legal nonprofits had the expertise to provide quality legal services but needed the partnership of strong and trusted community-based organizations to spread the word among their constituents. Members worked collaboratively to respond to service gaps, and there was no wrangling over funding or credit. According to Peter Pedemonti, executive director of the New Sanctuary Movement, "The DACA trainings have been essential for the immigrant community to get out real information that protects people from fraud. The sessions gave people the tools and confidence to apply for deferred action."

Accomplishments

P-DAN secured $75,000 of its 1-year budget of $111,700 and allocated these funds among partners. Most of the funds were used to support a part-time coordinator based at PICC. From August 2012 through August 2013, P-DAN members conducted 65 outreach events that reached 2,289 community members and 15 trainings that reached 333 providers, and they completed 373 applications. Additional funds secured in January

2014 enabled core partners PICC and HIAS Pennsylvania to continue the project on a more limited basis.

One of the first applicants in the region to benefit from DACA was J.S., a 30-year-old Bolivian national. J.S. was brought to the United States when he was 7 years old. He graduated from a magnet high school but despite his academic potential was unable to attend a 4-year college. At the time, he attended community college and was a computer specialist. He was also a leader in the immigrant rights movement. His DACA application was filed by the immigrant youth advocate at HIAS Pennsylvania. It was approved, and he obtained an employment authorization card. "To me, learning quenches my thirst; my dream is to attend college and become an engineer."

S.S., an Indonesian youth, had at the time lived in Philadelphia for almost half of his life; he attended Temple University, majoring in economics, and was being represented for a nominal fee by a private attorney: "DACA means opening doors of opportunity for me; I can now work legally in the U.S. and obtain a driver's license. But the most important thing of being granted DACA is not having to live in fear of being deported any longer. It surely takes a lot of weight off of your shoulders."

As with any coalition, especially one seeking to implement a new policy, P-DAN also encountered challenges. These included reaching isolated immigrant communities in the surrounding counties of Philadelphia and in rural areas as well as reaching diverse ethnic communities, especially those in which the issue of immigration status is not as openly discussed as it is in the Latino community, and forging partnerships with respected community organizations.

The application requirements were demanding. There was a major barrier to enrollment for individuals who met the age requirement and had lived in the United States for the requisite number of years but who did not yet meet the education requirement. Encouraging these young adults to enroll in a General Educational Development (GED) program to obtain a high school equivalency certificate, and finding a program to accept them, was an ongoing challenge. The application required significant documentation of age and confirmation of living in the United States. Many young immigrants were used to living a life of invisibility so as not to draw attention to their status and found it difficult to gather the evidence to meet these strict documentation requirements. Finally, the application fee of $465 was onerous for many of the unemployed young people.

DACA is certain to be around for the remainder of President Obama's administration, and it may become the foundation for a revitalized DREAM Act. The young immigrant activists, known as DREAMers, who courageously fought for the DREAM Act, are continuing their efforts to draw attention to their situation. PICC's work coordinating the P-DAN initiative helped the organization develop new and closer links with immigrant-serving and immigrants' rights organizations in the region while exploring with these groups a longer-term national policy solution for both young people and their families. P-DAN enabled us to test a cross-agency model that could be implemented in response to other immigration policy changes. Any organization interested in learning more about DACA or the work of the P-DAN coalition should contact Natasha Keleman at natashakeleman@paimmigrant.org or visit the PICC website at www.paimmigrant.org.

BUILDING A CULTURE OF COLLABORATION

Ashley Tobin

Getting started with the act of collaboration involves two key components: a group of willing participants and a structured conversation. Connecting Coffee is a free networking program for nonprofit professionals, started because there was no venue for people to describe their work, ask for what they needed, and form relationships with other agencies. In the structured environment of Connecting Coffee, a moderated small-group discussion, nonprofit professionals are coming together and solving problems.

We in the nonprofit sector tend to act as if there is a cold war among all the other agencies in our areas. We keep to ourselves and do not talk to other agencies; we only hear about their work from our donors or when those agencies get the big grant we wanted. We wonder how they are getting things done, but rarely do we ask them ourselves, and rarely do we truly understand who our competitors and our potential partners are.

This isolation can also contribute to staff turnover. The lack of a network of like-minded people increases the sense that you are the only one doing what you are doing. The ground-level work is hard, with an emotional investment that can take a toll on your key people. When a group of people starts talking about how hard it is, social bonds develop that make the next part of the conversation—finding solutions—easier. Some people have called this therapy for nonprofit professionals: It is not. It is a productive business tool that breaks down walls and creates pathways for communication and collaboration.

The greatest frustration in the nonprofit sector is when an agency creates a new program when a similar, high-quality program is already being offered by someone else. The act of partnering with another agency to share a program or expand its reach does not need to be a major undertaking. When agencies can identify their needs and then seek out partners to fill those needs with high-quality solutions, nonprofits become more efficient and more effective.

Connecting Coffee starts by building a common, shared interest. After we introduce ourselves, I ask a question to get the conversation started. If there is a specific topic for the session, the question will be about that topic. Sometimes we start with a question such as, "Who is doing great work in Philadelphia?" When I start with this question, very rarely is the answer "my agency," so we spend some time dissecting that.

The common feeling most often expressed is frustration. Having a chance to vent is an important part of the process, but because it is a moderated discussion, we do not dwell on the frustration for long. Instead, we start talking about solutions: What would change the shared frustration? What is a resource that you need to make this better?

In the fall of 2011, Philadelphia VIP hosted a Connecting Coffee about volunteer management, a topic that always gets a good cross-section of people at the table: executive directors, social workers, volunteer managers, development directors, and so on. The greater the diversity of voices, the better the conversation.

At this session, the group talked about how volunteer management can be a challenge because people who do not know how to manage volunteers, and who have job responsibilities outside of volunteer management, need to manage the work product and expectations of the volunteer and the person who is benefiting from the volunteer's efforts. Although they may be well meaning, volunteers do not always understand the beneficiary's situation, and their volunteer experiences can become frustrating.

For example, a lawyer who is helping a family through a legal problem may not understand why the family's phone works one day and not the next. That family might be on a prepaid cell phone plan and have run out of minutes. They might have needed to make some hard decisions about how to spend their money that month: food or phone? The lawyer may only see that he or she is having a hard time doing the pro bono work that will resolve the situation. The lawyer, the family, and the staff person are spending more time trying to manage the connection than they are in helping the family. Nonprofit professionals could come up with dozens of these examples; I use the lawyer example because there were representatives in the room from a number of agencies that work with lawyers.

The conversation then turned to solutions. What would make situations like these easier? After some deliberation, the group started talking about trying to find a shared resource for cultural competence training. They wanted a program that would show volunteers some of the realities they will find when they try to help. They wanted something engaging and interactive, something that could be provided in one session because so many volunteers do not have a lot of time to spend. The interactive training had to show the decisions that a family living in poverty needs to make. A short, persuasive video describing the life of such a family would be helpful and could be viewed anywhere.

The room was positively electric with the hope for a solution that would resolve this persistent and universal issue. I said I would do some research, and other people offered to reach out to organizations that they knew had well-developed volunteer training. For several months, I talked to video production companies, looked for funding, and talked to agencies that corral volunteers. And then I heard from the host of that day's session, Susan Wysor Nguema of Philadelphia VIP.

Philadelphia VIP is an agency that provides last-resort legal services for a low-income population, often helping people with basic needs such as shelter and health. In order to provide this legal help, they recruit and train lawyers, and Susan is one of those social workers who takes a project and runs with it. She talked to her leadership team, and they saw that this training program was within the mission and scope of the agency.

In October 2012, Philadelphia VIP held the first cultural competence training program—complete with continuing legal education credits in the coveted ethics category. Susan was invited to provide the same training to corporate in-house counsel at a large Philadelphia-based company. Her program is bridging gaps, misunderstandings, and hurt feelings between volunteers from the for-profit and nonprofit sectors. And she is doing it because the need and solution were identified at Connecting Coffee.

This example is, on a grand scale, what I see at Connecting Coffee each session: people articulating what they need and peers providing solutions.

It can be scary admitting that you need something, especially when you feel isolated. Many people who come to Connecting Coffee feel as if they are the only ones doing what they are doing, the only ones struggling. After we build that as a universal truth, we start getting to the productive discussions about solutions. People swap names of people who can help and available community resources and find new uses for existing resources. What about using free tickets to the theater as incentives for families that are starting to change the behaviors that landed them in difficult situations? Sure!

As Philadelphia nonprofit professionals start to have these conversations and see the benefits of collaboration, we are building the skills within the agencies to build partnerships instead of new programs and shared resources instead of secrets. Philadelphia and the people we serve are better for it, and in the future, we will have a system that is more effective and efficient because everyone is working together.

THE PHILADELPHIA REFUGEE HEALTH COLLABORATIVE

Gretchen Shanfeld

BACKGROUND

The Philadelphia Refugee Health Collaborative (PRHC) was established in 2008, under the leadership of Nationalities Service Center (NSC), to create an equitable system of refugee health care in the Philadelphia region. Consisting of eight refugee health clinics and three local refugee resettlement agencies, the Collaborative has made significant progress toward that goal. The Collaborative is a unique model of care for refugees in the United States. Key components of the model include close partnerships between resettlement agencies and medical providers, locations within large university health systems, and coordination between agencies. Since its inception, the Collaborative has increased its capacity for refugee screenings by over 220% (from 250 to 800 screenings annually).

Narrative

The Issue

Since the mid-1970s, large numbers of refugees have been resettled in the Philadelphia region; between 1983 and 2004, 33,000 refugees were resettled in the Delaware Valley. Currently, three local resettlement agencies—Nationalities Service Center, Lutheran Children and Family Service (LCFS), and HIAS—are resettling approximately 800 refugees to the region each year. Refugees typically come from many years of living in refugee camps or urban slums with limited access to health care, food, clean water, and hygiene. Many refugees arrive with unmanaged chronic health conditions and/or infectious diseases including heart disease, hypertension, tuberculosis (TB), and hepatitis. Refugees also experience emotional trauma resulting from war, displacement, and loss of loved ones and status, and they are frequently diagnosed with depression, anxiety, and posttraumatic stress disorder (PTSD). Eager to begin anew but struggling with limited English proficiency and limited understanding of the complex U.S. health care system, refugees need help navigating that system.

According to federal protocol, refugees must obtain a domestic health screening (immunizations and screening for TB, infectious diseases, parasites, and PTSD) and orientation to the U.S. health care system within 30 days of arrival. The screening process is typically facilitated by a state department of health or state refugee coordinator, but no such system exists in Pennsylvania. Until several years ago, local resettlement agencies struggled to find medical providers with the cultural competence and knowledge of refugee health needed to provide high-quality screenings and follow-up care. In the absence of coordinated partnerships with medical providers, resettlement agencies employed an ad hoc system of referring refugees to local private physicians and public health centers. However, those centers are so overburdened that it can take months to secure a screening appointment.

Best-Practice Research

The Centers for Disease Control publishes guidelines for screening recently arrived refugees (www.cdc.gov/immigrantrefugeehealth/guidelines/domestic/domestic-guidelines.html). These guidelines focus almost exclusively on the diagnosis and treatment of infectious diseases such as TB, lead exposure, and malaria. In recent years, increased discussion among medical providers who conduct refugee screenings has brought to light the need for more comprehensive screening, including for complex medical issues, mental health concerns, and chronic diseases including diabetes.

Furthermore, recent research on the patient-centered medical home movement is currently at the forefront of best practices in primary care medicine. This model utilizes the primary care office as the home base for patient care. By placing the PRHC clinics in large hospital systems with extensive access to specialized testing and specialty care, we are able to provide comprehensive health management to all refugees, particularly those with complex needs.

Case Study

In 2012, J.U., a 53-year-old refugee from Bhutan, arrived in Philadelphia. She had lived in a refugee camp in Nepal for over 20 years after being forced out of Bhutan. With limited access to medical care in her small village, J.U. was struck with rheumatic fever at an early age, and with only basic medical care available in the camp, she eventually developed rheumatic heart disease, which weakened her heart valves. She was unable to perform basic daily activities, and she was even so weak that she was unable to stand to cook dinner for her family. On her arrival in the United States, J.U. was screened by a partner PRHC clinic, where she was referred for an urgent cardiology appointment. Two weeks after her arrival, she was seen by cardiology within the hospital network, where she was referred for valve replacement surgery. She completed surgery 2 months after arrival and is now recovering at home, where for the first time in many years, she is able to walk without assistance. J.U. will be followed for ongoing care in the medical home at the PRHC clinic.

Partnership Model

In 2007, NSC and Jefferson Family Medicine Associations piloted a refugee health clinic model involving a close partnership between a resettlement agency and a medical provider. Since 2007, PRHC has led efforts to replicate and adapt this clinic model to establish additional refugee clinics in Philadelphia. Key elements of the refugee clinic model are:

- The medical provider establishes a weekly clinic dedicated to refugees.
- The medical provider and resettlement agency develop a scheduling and registration system and have regular biannual meetings to evaluate clinic functioning.
- The resettlement agency designates a staff person to function as the "clinic liaison" to escort new patients to the clinic, troubleshoot registration issues, complete immediate scheduling of follow-up specialist appointments, and help new patients fill prescriptions. The clinic liaison acts as the point person for communication with the clinic staff regarding patient care.
- The medical provider completes the required domestic health screening and provides immediate attention to chronic and acute health needs and ongoing primary care.
- The refugee clinic provides resident training in global health and cultural competence.
- Patients have access to an extensive network of specialty practices through the university health systems.

These clinics currently have the capacity to serve all incoming refugees, including 19 new adult patients and 14 new pediatric patients per week through the network of 8 clinics:

- Children's Hospital of Philadelphia—coordinated by HIAS

- Einstein Community Practice—coordinated by LCFS
- Einstein Pediatrics—coordinated by LCFS
- Drexel Women's Care Center—coordinated by NSC
- Fairmount Primary Care Center—coordinated by NSC
- Jefferson Family Medicine Associates—coordinated by NSC
- Nemours Pediatrics—coordinated by NSC
- Penn Center for Primary Care—coordinated by HIAS

Initially, new clinics formed in partnership with one specific resettlement agency. However, this meant that newly arrived refugees in Philadelphia did not have equal access to care. For example, until 2011, refugees resettled by LCFS were not connected with any of the refugee health clinics and were still receiving ad hoc referrals to community health centers. Since April 2012, all clinics accept regular referrals from all three resettlement agencies, resulting in a more equitable system of health care for all newly arriving refugees.

The PRHC has been funded in recent years by the Barra Foundation, which supports a coordinator who facilitates quarterly meetings among all partners, coordinates refugee health staff at the various resettlement agencies, and serves as a liaison between city and state departments of public health. The Collaborative meets formally on a quarterly basis to discuss best practices, challenges, and future opportunities. Additionally, clinicians and resettlement staff communicate daily to discuss challenging cases and share successes. It is important to note that the Collaborative does not provide funding above Medicaid reimbursements to clinicians; its success relies on a core network of champions at the eight provider clinics. Currently, the Collaborative is undergoing a strategic planning process to determine the future direction of the initiative.

Compared with 5 years ago, refugees arriving in Philadelphia are getting faster access to screenings, specialists, and primary care; more comprehensive and higher-quality screenings by physicians who specialize in refugee health; and targeted health education and support to enable their independent navigation of the health care system. From an original capacity of 250 new refugee patients per year in 2007, PRHC clinics now provide domestic health screenings; primary care (including newborns and pediatrics, adult medicine, and geriatric and obstetric and gynecological care); and access to laboratory, radiology, and subspecialty services to up to 800 newly arrived refugees each year as well as ongoing primary care for established patients and a specialized refugee women's health clinic.

THE TRANSFORMATIVE POSSIBILITIES OF NONPROFIT COLLABORATION

Annette Mattei

It may seem counterintuitive, but economic slowdowns are known to spark entrepreneurial ventures. A Kauffman Foundation study showed that more than half the companies on the 2009 *Fortune 500* list were launched during a recession or bear market, along with nearly half the firms on the 2008 *Inc.* list of America's fastest growing companies.

Nonprofits manifest similar urges toward reinvention when times are tough, and the tumult of the past decade has accelerated their cooperative and collaborative efforts. Recent trends underlying the accelerated collaboration in the nonprofit sector include:

- *Tremendous growth.* Between 2000 and 2008, the total number of nonprofits in the five counties of southeastern Pennsylvania grew by 36% (from 11,000 to 15,000). At the national level, nonprofits also experienced similar growth across every subsector.
- *Squeezed balance sheets.* The Nonprofit Finance Fund's (NFF) *2011 State of the Sector Survey* reported that roughly one third of responding nonprofits had a deficit, and 10% had "no cash." The Economy League of Greater Philadelphia reported similar findings for southeastern Pennsylvania.
- *Greater demand for services.* With the nation struggling with high unemployment, home foreclosures, and other tough economic conditions, 41% of the NFF's survey respondents said demand for their services had increased significantly in 2010, a trend in evidence since 2008.
- *Contracting budgets.* Most states are dramatically cutting programs in order to cover budget gaps. The Center for Budget and Policy

Priorities reported that despite stronger-than-expected state revenues for 2011, 42 states and the District of Columbia had to plug $103 billion in budget gaps for fiscal year 2012.

- *Sector contraction.* The IRS's recent decision to revoke the tax-exempt status of approximately 275,000 nonprofits for failing to file legally required annual reports will undoubtedly result in many nonprofits' merging together or even closing their doors.

The impact of these changes cannot be overstated. If the federal government accorded the nonprofit sector the same status it does other economic sectors (e.g., manufacturing), it would qualify as this region's third largest, with 242,000 employees who earn more than $11 billion in wages.

Innovating Through Collaboration

Collaboration among nonprofits can take many forms, from coordinated programming to full-fledged mergers. No one model is right for all nonprofits, but experts agree that successful collaborations are driven by the organizations' missions rather than by defensive reactions to external pressures. "Wise organizations choose strategic restructuring to further their missions," concluded La Piana Consulting, a firm specializing in nonprofit collaborations. "Saving money can be a result of strategic alliances and corporate integrations, but it is rarely the sole or even the primary reason…most often any 'savings' are plowed back into higher impact programs and services" ("Five Myths About Nonprofit Partnerships," www.lapiana.org/insights-for-the-sector/insights/collaboration-and-strategic-restructuring/five-myths.aspx).

As nonprofit collaborations grow in number, researchers have begun to mine the data and have arrived at some interesting observations:

- *Nonprofit collaboration does not necessarily mean mergers.* La Piana conducted an analysis of the applicants to the Lodestar Foundation's newly created Collaboration Prize and found that of the 175 highest-ranking applications, only 25% were actual mergers, whereas 50% involved joint programming, administrative consolidation, or some combination of both.

- *No one subsector dominates nonprofit collaboration.* La Piana's analysis also found that applicants represented every subsector of the nonprofit world.
- *Certain subsectors are more amenable to merger activity than others.* In a study of nonprofit merger filings made between 1996 and 2006 in four states (Massachusetts, Florida, Arizona, and North Carolina), the Bridgespan Group was able to identify the market characteristics of the subsectors that were amenable to nonprofit mergers. Merger-friendly subsectors tend to be large areas of concern served by many small organizations in which funding sources are impersonal (i.e., government as opposed to individual donations) that face major barriers to organic growth, such as government regulations. For example, the study cited child and family services as an example of a subsector that was humming with merger activity.
- *Nonprofits as a group are no more likely to merge than their for-profit counterparts; the exception is large organizations.* Bridgespan's study found that the cumulative merger rate for nonprofits was essentially the same as that for for-profits: 1.5% versus 1.7%. The vast majority of mergers—nonprofit and for-profit—are between small organizations and companies. However, the merger rate for large nonprofits (i.e., those with budgets of at least $50 million) is one-tenth that for large for-profits. Bridgespan attributes this disparity to the difference in incentives. For-profit mergers are driven by financial incentives, particularly payouts to individual parties and fees paid to third-party "matchmakers." Nonprofit mergers, in the best of circumstances, are strategic decisions driven by organizations' missions; theoretically, it is the community as a whole, not individual parties, that benefits.

Our understanding of nonprofit collaboration will surely expand in the coming years as organizations continue to explore new ways of operating in persistently difficult economic conditions and with increasing demand for their services. The entrance of new intermediaries such as the Lodestar Foundation's Collaboration Prize and

Boston's Catalyst Fund is likely to help step up the pace of nonprofit collaboration.

Furthermore, research initiatives such as the Arizona, Indiana, and Michigan (AIM) Alliance, a Lodestar-supported project involving universities in these three states will offer new insight into nonprofit collaboration and identify effective models and best practices that will be relevant to our own region's nonprofits.

In the not-too-distant future, we may look back on this period and realize it was a time of entrepreneurial innovation among nonprofits as they collaborated in new and transformative ways.

5

Collaboration Case Studies

Taz Hussein, Patricia Hampson Eget,
Russell Johnson, William P. Brown, Jr.,
Robert M. Gallagher, Will Gonzalez,
and Suzan Neiger Gould

EDITORS' OVERVIEW

Chapter 4 looked at a few Philadelphia collaborations with a slight emphasis on the partnerships themselves but with more of a focus on the beneficiaries of the various collaborative efforts. Chapter 5 gets into more detail about how some partnerships themselves happened, including what has made them work. The YMCA of the USA's partnership with UnitedHealth Group (UHG) was particularly innovative, and it was based on sound principles that can effectively guide even the most informal partnership efforts.

THE FUTURE OF HEALTH CARE IS HERE: PARTNERSHIPS WITH COMMUNITY-BASED ORGANIZATIONS

Taz Hussein

The poor man who enters into a partnership with one who is rich makes a risky venture.

—Titus Maccius Plautus

In 2009, YMCA of the USA (the Y) and UHG formed what would turn out to be a historic partnership. Under the terms of this agreement, UHG would reimburse the Y for each of its eligible insured customers who successfully participated in the YMCA's Diabetes Prevention Program (DPP). This program targets individuals with prediabetes— the precursor to the disease—and aims to help them lose at least 5% of their body weight. Research has shown that participants who achieve this goal reduce their risk of developing type 2 diabetes by almost 60% (Diabetes Prevention Program Research Group, 2002).

Over the past few years, UHG has invested millions of dollars in its partnership with the Y. To my knowledge, this partnership represents one of the first times that a commercial health insurance payer has contracted with a social services community-based organization (CBO) to offer a chronic disease prevention program on a true pay-for-performance basis. Partnerships like these represent the future of health care, and this section of the chapter explores what is driving the formation of these partnerships and what it will take for them to succeed over the long term.

BACKGROUND

As described more fully in "Using National Networks to Tackle Chronic Disease" (Hussein & Kerrissey, 2013), the Y's DPP is a year-long program. Participants meet for 1 hour per week for the first 16 weeks and then monthly for another 8 months. The sessions are conducted in a small-group format, usually with anywhere from 8 to 15 participants, and are led by trained lifestyle coaches. At each session, participants learn about healthy eating habits and discuss their own impediments to changing their eating and physical activity behaviors.

In approximately the fifth week, participants are also encouraged to start incorporating 150 minutes per week of physical activity into their lives. The DPP is considered an evidence-based intervention, and it was adapted from a similar program developed through extensive research by academics and funded by the National Institutes of Health (Ackermann & Marrero, 2007).

The Y is the national office that supports a federated network of approximately 900 independent, local Y associations across the country. UHG is a more-than-$80 billion diversified health and well-being company that, among its other businesses, provides health insurance to tens of millions. UHG entered into this partnership in part because it was attracted by Y's ability to achieve the same weight loss results as clinical providers but at much lower costs. With thousands of sites located across the country, the Y also offered the benefit of being a service provider with tremendous scale. Importantly, however, UHG could develop this partnership by negotiating with one national office rather than up to 900 legally separate entities.

The Forces That Drive Partnerships Among CBOs, Health Care Providers, and Payers

Tectonic shifts are underway in the field of health care. The decades-old paradigm of "more"—more hospitals, more specialists and surgeons, more (and usually more expensive) treatments, and more access to high-end technology—is giving way to a renewed emphasis on maintaining health, preventing disease, and obtaining primary care. The rationale for these shifts is clear: By almost all measures, the United States spends more on health care than any other developed country, and yet our citizens are sicker than most and have shorter life expectancies (Woolf & Aron, 2013).

We have arrived at this point, in large measure, as a result of how we finance health care. The health care system has been incentivized to treat sickness rather than maintain health. The results are well known: Health care expenditures now account for almost 18% of gross domestic product (GDP), and Medicare and Medicaid, which consume an ever-larger share of state and federal budgets, crowd out other worthwhile investments in education and infrastructure. And many of us feel the pain as our health care premiums and out-of-pocket costs increase by double digits each year.

With the Patient Protection and Affordable Care Act (ACA) now firmly the law of the land and any meaningful debt reduction package likely to include changes in entitlement programs, health care financing mechanisms are changing rapidly. Commercial insurers, and even Medicaid, are experimenting again with global payment schemes: paying health care providers a fixed amount annually to take care of a group of insured customers or covered beneficiaries. At the heart of all of these initiatives is an attempt to promote improved health outcomes at a lower cost.

Attempts to put the nation on sounder financial footing for the long term are also causing tremors in the world of CBOs that provide social services. A vast array of nonprofits that provide substance abuse, mental health, housing, and a host of other critical services to some of our nation's most vulnerable populations has historically operated alongside, but largely at the periphery of, our health care system. Massive cuts in public funding, the primary source of financial support for most of these organizations, have already pushed some of them to close their doors and are pushing many others to pursue mergers and other types of strategic collaborations.

We Are Just at the Beginning of a New Wave of Partnerships

Given the changes buffeting the worlds of health care and social services CBOs, we are seeing more serious discussions of partnerships between CBOs and the health care sector than ever before. We are not referring here to short-term arrangements between a clinical provider and a social services nonprofit to collaboratively offer a program in response to a specially funded initiative, but rather to health care providers who are formally integrating networks of CBOs into their care delivery systems, and to payers who view social service CBOs as reimbursable providers of services that were previously the sole purview of highly degreed clinicians.

Examples of these partnership discussions and constructs, while all still generally at early stages, are beginning to proliferate. A few months ago, I participated in a meeting organized by the Administration on Community Living and the SCAN Foundation that focused explicitly on the kinds of technical assistance needed to support aging and disability service networks in becoming more effective partners with health care organizations. Leaders from the participating nonprofits were eager to understand how they could position their organizations to establish formal partnerships with health care entities. In a similar vein, the Alliance for Children and Families—an international membership association representing 350 human service agencies—is very actively promoting to health care providers and payers the role that its member agencies can play in addressing the needs of the "5/50" population (i.e., the 5% of Medicaid beneficiaries who account for 50% of Medicaid's total expenditures).

What Will It Take for These Partnerships to Be Successful Over the Long Term?

Partnerships can be tricky business. For partnerships between CBOs and health care providers or payers to be successful over the long term, both parties must be clear about their own interests, their assessment of what the other party brings to the table, and why working together is better than working alone.

Consider the partnership between the Y and UHG. The 160-year-old Y is a mission-driven organization that seeks, among other things, to help individuals and families improve their health. It tries to reach as many people as it can with proven programs such as the DPP. Prior to joining forces with UHG, the Y had relied primarily on government funding to support the rollout of the program to about 30 locations, but public funding, while critical to getting the program off the ground, would never have been enough to help it achieve meaningful scale. In addition to direct financial support, UHG offered the Y access to a large pool of potential program participants and the ability to develop critical program infrastructure, including a system that allows the Y to monitor the results of program participants across the country in real time and to collect reimbursement from any third-party payer.

UHG provides health insurance coverage to tens of millions of people. It collects premiums from its insured customers, both individuals and companies, and agrees to pay for medical costs incurred by those customers. For every one of its insured customers who develops a disease such as diabetes, UHG must pay for treatment, which often costs thousands of dollars annually. For UHG, the DPP offered a way to prevent or delay the onset of an expensive and debilitating disease among its customers. In the Y, UHG found a partner that could offer a high-quality version of this intervention practically everywhere UHG had customers. And, not insignificantly, UHG could form this partnership by negotiating with a small number of people in the Y's national office rather than representatives from several hundred independent legal entities.

Clearly, there are many reasons to recommend the development of mutually beneficial partnerships between CBOs and health care providers or payers; the devil is in the details. CBOs considering these types of partnerships should start by asking themselves if they can:

- Quantify and communicate the value their services will bring to a health care provider or payer in terms that matter to them (e.g., cost avoidance or additional revenue generation)
- Price their services such that the value they provide exceeds what is charged
- Develop a sustainable operating structure for their services such that variable costs are less than the price charged
- Secure funding to build the infrastructure to deliver high-quality services
- Effectively monitor service delivery to ensure that it is of the highest quality and complies with appropriate regulations (e.g., the Health Insurance Portability and Accountability Act)

While the initial impetus for many of these partnership discussions may be the big environmental shifts noted earlier, the best of the partnerships that ultimately form will be much less about a path to survival for the partnering organizations and more about a way for them to better serve their target beneficiaries. For health care providers and payers, these partnerships offer an opportunity to actually improve the health of the individuals and families they serve rather than just treating them when they are sick, and to do so cost-effectively. For CBOs, these partnerships may allow them to secure more sustainable sources of funding for their work and to scale up and serve far more beneficiaries than they may have previously imagined possible.

STRENGTHENING PROGRAMS AND SERVICES FOR IMMIGRANT SENIORS IN CHALLENGING ECONOMIC TIMES

Patricia Hampson Eget

Elderly immigrants are among southeastern Pennsylvania's most vulnerable residents, and providing cost-effective culturally and linguistically targeted services for this population is a pressing challenge facing nonprofits in the Philadelphia region. Southeastern Pennsylvania's Asian population increased by 58% in the past 10 years according to U.S. census data, much faster than the 5% growth in the region's population. The Asian American community's demographic expansion tells a story of vibrant, growing communities, but accompanied by a corresponding increase in the needs of the most vulnerable, particularly the elderly.

Asian seniors are more likely than other seniors to face language and cultural barriers in accessing needed social services including health information, public benefits, housing, social and recreation activities, and transportation. While overall, only 12% of seniors in the United States are immigrants, 81% of Asian seniors are foreign born. Additionally, 60% of Asian seniors report speaking English "less than well" compared with 8% of all seniors, and 12.5% live below the poverty line compared with 10% of seniors nationwide (Asian American Federation, 2009). Asian seniors are thus more likely than others to encounter linguistic and social isolation and to live in poverty.

Despite the Asian American community's growth, few senior centers, government agencies, or other social service agencies in the region have the linguistic and cultural skills necessary to meet the needs of Asian seniors. Additionally, the nonprofits that serve these seniors in the region are often fragmented and lack the financial resources to offer them high-quality services.

This section explores how two strategic alliances between nonprofits that served the Asian American community expanded their linguistically and culturally targeted programming for Asian seniors. Penn Asian Senior Services (PASSi), Pennsylvania's first and largest nonprofit home care agency for Asian seniors, entered a strategic alliance with the Korean Senior Association of Greater Philadelphia (KSAGP) to better serve Korean seniors.

PASSi has established trust between southeastern Pennsylvania's Korean community and its 13 bilingual, skilled administrative staff who support the programming for Korean seniors. PASSi's mission is to support the well-being of ailing Asian American seniors who are disadvantaged by language and cultural barriers, and 100% of the seniors PASSi serves are low income. PASSi currently provides home care to 393 frail, elderly Asian Americans, approximately 100 of whom are Korean.

KSAGP is a nonprofit organization led by Korean seniors that was founded in 1971 to meet the needs of Philadelphia's growing number of elderly Koreans who were struggling to adapt to life in the United States with limited financial resources. With more than 60 active members, KSAGP offers weekly programming that educates seniors about American culture and improves their English skills; organizes interactive workshops on a variety of health, civic, and social topics; and offers free music and dancing classes.

KSAGP initially relied on donations from small Korean-owned businesses to fund its operations. Since the 2008 recession, KSAGP has found it difficult to raise funds for its weekly senior programming from the local Korean business community. Additionally, KSAGP lacks any paid staff, and its leadership speaks limited English; the organization thus lacks the administrative capacity to secure other funding streams and is not equipped to meet the growing demand for programs for low-income Korean seniors in Philadelphia.

PASSi and KSAGP secured a $20,000 Targeted Investment Grant from United Way of Greater Philadelphia and Southern New Jersey to fund a strategic alliance that would focus on joint programming for Korean seniors. PASSi and KSAGP share the goal of assisting English-limited Korean seniors in Philadelphia and have a long history of collaboration. The United Way funding allowed the organizations to expand an existing partnership and create a strategic alliance that has increased the capacity of both organizations to serve Korean seniors.

KSAGP now has access to PASSi's bilingual administrative staff and the capacity to pursue diverse funding streams. The strategic alliance has increased KSAGP's administrative efficiency and the quality of its senior programming while still allowing Korean seniors themselves to lead the association. This saves KSAGP money and allows the group to allocate its limited financial resources to programming rather than overhead and salary expenses.

KSAGP and PASSi's joint programming and strategic alliance proved extremely successful during the partnership's first 6 months. Before PASSi and KSAGP created their strategic alliance and joint programming, approximately 20 Korean seniors attended KSAGP's weekly program. PASSi and KSAGP started offering weekly joint programming in mid-September 2012. By the end of December of the same year, nearly 60 Korean seniors attended the weekly programs, a 300% increase in attendance.

Additionally, PASSi and KSAGP have qualitative evidence that Korean seniors are extremely satisfied with the improved programming. The strategic alliance has allowed PASSi and KSAGP to move the programming location from KSAGP's office in northeast Philadelphia on Rising Sun Avenue to *Hankuk Daily News*'s Cheltenham office. KSAGP's office lacked space for exercise programming, was poorly maintained, and was inconvenient to public transportation. *Hankuk Daily News*'s office is located close to public transportation and Philip Murray House, a large senior housing complex with a significant concentration of Korean residents. PASSi and KSAGP used the larger facility to add line dancing, a popular activity with Korean seniors, as an important part of the program. This provides a fun way for the seniors to remain physically fit.

In addition to finding a better location, KSAGP and PASSi leveraged the strategic alliance to enhance the quality of programming. Previously, KSAGP only had limited funds for refreshments and usually ordered pizza. Pizza has poor nutritional value and is not especially appetizing to Korean seniors, who strongly prefer Korean food. KSAGP and PASSi used their shared resources to purchase Korean lunch boxes for all attendees. These lunch boxes feature a choice of sautéed beef, chicken, or pork, fish, rice, and vegetables prepared Korean style. This hot, nutritious meal is a very important benefit for these seniors, who are often too old to cook for themselves and have limited means to purchase healthy food.

PASSi leveraged its strong community connections to enhance the senior program content. Its administrative staff worked with KSAGP to identify topics of interest to Korean seniors and then secured Korean experts in those particular topics. Topics discussed at the weekly program include information about common diseases, nutrition, senior housing and transportation resources, the Access card for seniors, how to obtain American citizenship, personal safety in Philadelphia, acupuncture, herbal medicines, Korean versus American art, music, and culture, and many other topics.

Equally important, the strategic alliance increased interest among other Koreans in volunteering to help with KSAGP and PASSi's weekly senior program. The program now has three Korean volunteers who assist with logistics, publicity, and other items, and these volunteers will help the program remain sustainable over the long term by reducing staff costs.

PASSi and KSAGP's strategic alliance and joint senior programming demonstrated the positive impact of strategic alliances in expanding programming for elderly immigrants while still allowing them to have a strong voice in that programming. Elderly immigrants often remain overlooked, vulnerable members of southeastern Pennsylvania's senior population. Nonprofit organizations should look for innovative, cost-effective ways to meet the growing needs of these seniors. Strategic alliances can reduce administrative and overhead costs and allow nonprofits to devote more resources to programming and direct services.

NORTH PENN COMMONS: FOSTERING SOCIAL INNOVATION THROUGH COLLABORATION

Russell Johnson, William P. Brown, Jr., Robert M. Gallagher, and Suzan Neiger Gould

Four nonprofit organizations in the North Penn community of Montgomery County—Advanced Living Communities (ALC, a developer of affordable senior housing), Manna on Main Street (a soup kitchen and food pantry), North Penn YMCA, and PEAK Center (a senior center)—have developed an innovative partnership, now known as the North Penn Commons, to colocate their facilities on a shared campus in Lansdale, Pennsylvania. By sharing facilities and resources, the partners intend to collaborate on programs, provide better access to services, and use financial and volunteer resources most effectively.

Their collaboration promises to strengthen the capacity of each of the partners and create a vibrant community center at the eastern gateway to Lansdale Borough. The project's design fully supports the goals of Lansdale Borough's community development and revitalization plans. The North Penn Community Health Foundation (NPCHF), an independent, private foundation, has supported the collaboration through strategic funding for visioning and organizational, legal, and fundraising planning and support as well as collaborative program development.

The Genesis of the Collaboration

Since its founding in 2002, NPCHF has sought to address select health and human service problems and needs in the North Penn area and surrounding Montgomery County. The foundation combines high-impact grant making with capacity building for area nonprofits. Partnerships and collaborations are fostered and encouraged to promote learning and creative problem solving and to leverage the core competencies and resources of collaborators who seek to address unmet community needs.

As part of a broad community needs assessment, the foundation joined with other public and private funders to commission the 2006 BoomerANG Project ("Boomers—Aging's Next Generation"), which highlighted the explosive growth of the 55- to 64-year-old cohort in Montgomery County, and found that these "boomers" seek a different set of services and choices than are currently offered by traditional senior centers; they want more focus on health and wellness provided in a setting that allows for intergenerational connections. The study also found that quality, affordable housing—especially for low-income seniors—is almost nonexistent in the region and that those units that do exist have long waiting lists (Marcus & Migliaccio, 2006).

Recognizing these challenges, each of the four partner organizations had planned to expand and update their individual facilities to better serve their constituents. As a funder of each of the organizations, NPCHF brought the leaders of the agencies together to discuss a potential collaboration. After a series of facilitated meetings, it became clear that developing a shared campus would enhance the opportunities of each organization to achieve its mission in the most cost-effective way *and*, by virtue of their working at the same site, foster opportunities to collaborate on new programs to enrich the lives of their existing constituents and attract new ones as well.

As a business located in the North Penn Commons, each organization maintains its autonomy and independent governance but agrees to share certain operating and maintenance functions for the campus. The partners have executed legal joint venture agreements that define the rights and responsibilities of each organization in this collaborative venture.

The Shared Campus

With the addition of the 3-acre property adjacent to the Y's current 8-acre campus, the new 11-acre campus on East Main Street will include 60 independent living units for low-income seniors situated on three floors above the Manna and PEAK offices and program facilities; a commercial kitchen designed to support the culinary needs of all four partners; an expanded Y that will include a zero-entry family pool, a new gymnasium, locker rooms, and classroom and community spaces; and a lobby atrium that will serve as a shared gathering space for all members, clients, volunteers, and community residents. The site is situated in a walkable downtown business community, is served by a public transportation bus route and nearby rail service, and has accessible parking.

The partner organizations will share certain construction costs including land development, architectural fees, and site work. Because the project includes affordable senior housing, it qualified for support through Low Income Housing Tax Credits, a federal tax credit program administered by the Pennsylvania Housing Finance Agency (PHFA) that awarded $11.3 million in tax credits through a highly competitive process. PHFA also bestowed its first-ever design award to the North Penn Commons project in recognition of its unique strengths. Thanks to this unique funding formula, the completed facility will be larger and more robust than any that the partners could have built separately. The partners are coordinating fundraising through a single campaign, One Four All, that is seeking potential donors to make gifts to the collaborative campaign—knowing that their single gift will benefit four worthy nonprofits and thousands of community residents. During the capital campaign, each partner has agreed to collaborate on and coordinate annual giving campaigns to help educate potential donors on the need for both annual giving and capital support for this unique opportunity.

Construction started in spring 2014, and the campus is expected to be completed by fall 2015. Once the campus opens, it will operate as a condominium association, with the partners sharing common operating expenses such as housekeeping, landscaping, maintenance, security, and insurance. This cost sharing will mitigate the effect of any increased operating costs, freeing more resources for community services rather than overhead.

Leveraging Collaboration

While the building plan breaks new ground in this community, the opportunities for service collaboration are even more powerful. For example:

- The partners plan to leverage Manna's expertise in food preparation to benefit each organization while generating additional revenue for Manna. The shared lobby café will be supported by a commercial kitchen operated by Manna staff and volunteers. Multiple generations will enjoy connecting with each other around a meal. Manna staff will provide snacks to the Y's child care programs and full lunches for PEAK Center's congregant meal program. A small convenience store will also sell staples such as bread and milk to ALC residents and other visitors.
- Volunteers are essential to the operation of each of the partner's facilities—Manna on Main Street has 1,200 active volunteers and a waiting list. Manna purchased a robust volunteer management and scheduling software tool that will centralize volunteer

management—including recruitment, orientation, and scheduling—through Manna on behalf of all its partners. Within the collaboration, current volunteers will be exposed to new volunteer opportunities. These same volunteers also represent potential new members for North Penn Y, PEAK Center, and ALC.

- ALC residents and Manna clients and volunteers will be encouraged to use the fitness programs offered by YMCA and the PEAK Center, with financial assistance available as needed. The PEAK Center will offer social services and counseling to Manna's senior clients.
- The partners will take a coordinated approach to event planning, such as avoiding date conflicts for important events, coordinating space scheduling, and utilizing volunteer resources to assist in setup and management. All of the partners regularly invite community organizations to their respective sites. In the new facility, partners will have enhanced opportunities to offer services, education, and support as a secondary benefit to the community's nonprofits and businesses.
- Shared transportation services will bring clients and members to the campus, increasing participation and reducing isolation.
- Innovative collaborative programs will offer the partners new opportunities for grant funding, building capacity for the future.

While construction is underway, the partners have been planning how they will approach joint decision making, program planning, and community outreach and engagement by inviting residents, members, clients, and the broader community to share their experiences, ideas, and hopes with the goal of further developing the power of collaboration. They established a chief executive officer (CEO) council, currently chaired by the executive director of Manna, to ensure regular, structured communication about operating challenges and programming opportunities.

During the planning process and construction, new opportunities are already taking form. For instance, PEAK closed and sold its old facility and relocated its programs to an ALC campus, and during the first week of operation at the new site, community participation in the noontime congregant meal program more than doubled. Manna relocated to a larger facility in April 2012 and is using its new commercial kitchen equipment and culinary expertise to enhance its own programming in preparation for the expanded role it will have on the new campus. PEAK has contracted with the Y to use its staff to provide fitness programs. Best of all, the leadership of the partner organizations continue to ask questions and explore new opportunities that are contributing to an understanding of how to efficiently leverage time, resources, and talents to best address community needs and interests.

While each partner will benefit from the economies of scale and cost-sharing opportunities this collaboration will provide, the project has the potential to dramatically improve how clients of each of the four partner organizations—ALC, Manna on Main Street, North Penn YMCA, and PEAK Center—receive services and interact with their neighbors. The North Penn Commons is an innovative model that seeks to capitalize on the strengths each partner brings and to build community by offering a range of much-needed services in a central location. The North Penn Community Health Foundation is proud to be a funder of this unique partnership.

THE LATINO VOTER ID WORK GROUP:
A CASE STUDY OF COLLABORATIVE LEADERSHIP
IN PHILADELPHIA'S BARRIO

Will Gonzalez

Ceiba, a coalition of four Latino nonprofits in Philadelphia, used collaborative leadership principles to coalesce 20 organizations to turn concern about the potential of Pennsylvania's voter ID law to suppress voting in the Hispanic community into a catalyst to promote voter registration and turnout. This collaborative leadership encouraged dialogue, promoted trust, and fostered a sense of ownership of the collective's work among the participating organizations in the group. The cooperative effort helped the organizations focus on results instead of on who got the credit. It furthermore made clear that Ceiba's role was to provide leadership of the collaborative process rather than leadership of the group. Collaborative leadership served the Latino community well not only because it helped to tackle a serious threat but also because it demonstrated its potential to nurture future collaborations.

On March 12, 2012, one of the most restrictive voter ID measures in the nation became law in Pennsylvania. The law mandated that voters in the Keystone State present identification every time they vote, and limited the forms of ID that were acceptable at the polls. Proponents praised the law as a tool to prevent voter fraud. Opponents considered it a vehicle to suppress the voting rights of people who have difficulty securing acceptable forms of ID.

On May 1, 2012, the Public Interest Law Center of Philadelphia, the Advancement Project, the American Civil Liberties Union (ACLU) of Pennsylvania, and the Washington, DC, law firm of Arnold & Porter LLP filed a lawsuit in the Commonwealth Court of Pennsylvania to overturn the law. After several hearings, court decisions, and appeals, Commonwealth Court Judge Bernard L. McGinley issued an order on January 17, 2014, that permanently blocked the controversial photo identification law on the grounds that it unconstitutionally disenfranchised large numbers of voters. Judge McGinley reaffirmed his opinion on April 28, 2014, when he denied the Commonwealth's motion to reconsider his earlier ruling. On May 8, 2014, Governor Tom Corbett announced that the Commonwealth would not appeal the court's ruling, thus ending the implementation of the law.

Although litigation was eventually successful, never was there a guarantee that a court challenge by itself would stop the law from going into effect. Over the last few years, 34 states have passed laws requiring voters to show some form of identification at the polls. As of May 8, 2014, 31 of these voter identification laws are in force according to the National Conference of State Legislatures (www.ncsl.org/research/elections-and-campaigns/voter-id.aspx). Groups concerned about the deleterious effects of the voter ID law in Pennsylvania had to prepare for the worst in case the court challenge failed.

Latinos, specifically Puerto Ricans, were one of the voting groups most adversely affected by the law. One reason for this is the Department of Homeland Security's 2010 ruling that invalidated birth certificates issued to people born before July 1, 2010, in Puerto Rico, a U.S. island territory in the Caribbean. Puerto Ricans of voting age can no longer use their original birth certificates to obtain driver's licenses or photo identification; they must now acquire entirely new birth certificates. Long queues, an inefficient online application system, and poor record keeping make procuring new birth certificates from the Puerto Rican government a difficult process.

Sixty-five percent of the more than 187,000 Latinos who live in the Philadelphia area are Puerto Rican. The voter ID law appeared destined to suppress voting in the city's Latino community.

Latino nonprofit organizations concerned about the erosion of voting rights in their community during a presidential election sought to take action to help people comply with the law. Some of them joined the Committee of Seventy's nonpartisan PA Voter ID Coalition, but they soon realized that a more focused, community-based approach was needed.

In July 2012, Associación de Puertorriqueños en Marcha, Concilio de Organizaciones Hispanas de Filadelfia (Concilio), Congreso de Latinos Unidos, Esperanza, the Hispanic Bar Association, and the National Council of La Raza joined forces and utilized Ceiba as a convener and lead organization to develop the Latino Voter ID Work Group. Ceiba is a coalition of four organizations in the Latino community: Concilio, Esperanza, Finanta, and the Norris Square Civic Association.

The Latino Voter ID Work Group became an affiliated subgroup of the PA Voter ID Coalition and aggressively recruited other Hispanic organizations to be part of the effort. Over the course of the summer and fall, the group successfully:

- Helped people understand, in English and Spanish, the voter ID law by organizing more than 30 presentations in community settings, discussing the issue in the media, and carrying out door-to-door outreach in more than 30 political divisions in predominantly Hispanic neighborhoods
- Equipped community-based organizations in the barrio with information and tools related to the voter ID law and voting rights by organizing staff trainings and preparing resource guides
- Assisted voters with challenges they faced in obtaining their IDs by organizing birth certificate legal clinics, assisting people at the Pennsylvania Department of Transportation, and referring people to the appropriate agencies or legal services organizations to resolve their issues

These activities reduced the confusion about the law generated by litigation, the mixed messages and often-confusing policies of the state, and the malicious or misguided efforts of some political action groups.

Collaborative leadership was instrumental in the work group's success. The group organized regular meetings, encouraged inclusiveness, ensured participants the opportunity to be heard, and quickly addressed conflicts and disputes within the group.

The focus on facts over feelings, nurtured by the collaborative leadership, helped to address disputes. When conflicts did arise, the organizations that were presenting divergent points of view were encouraged to bring more information to the table and to work together to help the collective make decisions based on their findings. Requests for additional information also quelled the occasional gadfly who participated at a single meeting and tried to subvert the process.

Collaborative leadership was able to help the work group carry out its activities despite limited material resources. Using the mantra of "we don't want to reinvent the wheel," the group relied on existing materials and partners' experience with particular activities. For example, instead of issuing its own flyers or informational materials about the voter ID law, the group embraced those created by the PA Voter ID Coalition and the ACLU. The emphasis was on the integrity of these materials in terms of information, and on the quality of the translations, not on whose logo was on the heading.

Motivating partners toward effectiveness after they had committed to carry out an activity was achieved by the collaborative leadership principle of developing small teams of fellow partners to plan, report, reevaluate, and implement each task. The partner that made the commitment was primarily responsible for the activity but was not left alone to bear the brunt of the planning. This approach was useful even with prominent and experienced work group partners. For example, in the midst of planning the birth certificate legal clinics, the partner that had committed to undertaking the activity had to attend to important organizational responsibilities including participation at a vital out-of-state conference. The partner had been responsible for organizing birth certificate legal clinics in previous years but was now tasked with organizing two clinics in seven days that aimed to serve a large number of people. Having a team plan the clinics allowed the partner to attend to its other responsibilities while work group teammates continued organizing the event. The clinics thus took place in a timely and efficient manner.

In terms of the media, the work group coordinated but did not try to control the messages or the exposure of its partners. The media spotlight has been known to generate jealousies within groups and detract from the positive work being done. Partners were free to speak to the press if they so desired, and their work was highlighted when the work group scheduled media events. Collaborative leadership, however, requires that the convener or lead organization subordinate its ego. When the work group organized its biggest voter ID press conference, Ceiba limited its role to simply introducing the speakers. The partners made the substantive presentations, addressed media questions, and fulfilled subsequent requests for additional comments after the conference.

A strategic planning process over the previous winter and spring had prepared Ceiba to use collaborative leadership principles during the following summer and fall. During that planning, Ceiba's board, staff, and stakeholders reached a consensus that the organization needed to significantly augment its advocacy efforts. Protecting the community's voting rights was connected in many ways to Ceiba's updated mission: promoting the economic development and financial inclusion of Philadelphia's Latino community through collaborations and advocacy aimed at ensuring their access to quality housing.

The strategic plan called for Ceiba to coalesce community organizations around advocacy efforts without requiring the administrative procedures of membership. Ceiba is on a course to amend its bylaws accordingly and eliminate the membership structure entirely; it is turning instead to collaborative leadership principles to guide its advocacy work.

It is almost impossible for any individual or organization to address today's complex socioeconomic challenges alone. The growing size and diversity of the Hispanic community, however, present Latino organizations with great opportunities to confront challenges in a collective way.

The implementation of the voter ID law was eventually stopped through litigation. However, collaborative leadership did more than just prepare the Latino community for a worst-case scenario: It showed a productive way for Latino organizations to collectively address community problems and cultivated a renewed willingness to work cooperatively for a common purpose.

The Community Tool Box of the University of Kansas is right when it says that collaborative leadership breeds more collaborative leadership and that more collaboration leads to exploring novel ways to solve problems.

REFERENCES

Ackermann, R. T., & Marrero, D. G. (2007). Adapting the Diabetes Prevention Program lifestyle intervention for delivery in the community: The YMCA model. *The Diabetes Educator, 33*(1), 69, 74–75, 77.

Asian American Federation. (2009). *Profile of Asian American seniors in the United States*. Retrieved from www.aafny.org/cic/briefs/usseniors2009 .pdf

Diabetes Prevention Program Research Group. (2002). Reduction in the incidence of type 2 diabetes with lifestyle intervention or metformin. *The New England Journal of Medicine 346*(6), 393–403. doi: 10.1056/ NEJMoa012512

Hussein, T., & Kerrissey, M. (2013). Using national networks to tackle chronic disease. *Stanford Social Innovation Review, 11*(1). Retrieved from www.ssireview.org/articles/entry/using_national_networks_to_ tackle_chronic_disease

Marcus, M., & Migliaccio, J. (2006). *BoomerANG Project Montgomery County, Pennsylvania*. Colmar, PA: North Penn Community Health Foundation (NPCHF). Retrieved from http://npchf.org/sites/npchf.org/files/ attachments/boomerang_report_sunflowers_0.pdf

Woolf, S. H., & Aron, L. (Eds.). (2013). *U.S. health in international perspective: Shorter lives, poorer health*. Washington, DC: National Academies Press.

6

Joint Ventures in the Social Sector

Nicholas D. Torres

INTRODUCTION

Joint ventures present an exciting opportunity for organizations and individuals to partner. This chapter lays out multiple joint venture partnerships and legal templates.

A joint venture can take many forms and be formal or informal, but the underlying principle of its success or failure starts with the person or people with whom you will be doing business. Any organization exploring a joint venture should walk into a partnership with the following partnership questions:

1. What are the benefits (social, financial, competitive advantage, etc.) of forming or entering into a partnership?
2. What is the other organization and/or person's motivation for partnering? Is it genuine and aligned with my organization's own motivation and mission?
3. Do I like the person or people I will be working with in this potential partnership? Can I trust them?

Assuming there is a benefit, the motivation is clear, and you think you can trust the person(s), the next step is to analyze the financial and business prospective alignments and benefits and the potential legal arrangement between the two organizations that are pursuing the venture. A successful and sustainable partnership requires that the benefits and controls for each respective organization be stated early and clearly defined. Based on how each organization defines its respective financial and legal goals, the joint venture will develop into one of three types:

- *Marriage*: An equal partnership in which both organizations share the benefits and risks and in which, if a separation occurs, the initiative dies or both parties have equal say in the terms of the separation.
- *Parent/child*: An agreement in which one organization has formally agreed to support another organization's launch, motivated by the potential for social impact and an understanding that nothing is owed to the parent organization.
- *Prenuptial*. An agreement in which one organization ultimately has legal, governance, or financial control of the initiative and, when desired, can move forward independently.

This chapter discusses four joint venture case studies comprising their inceptions, launches, and life spans, with two ending in the termination of the venture and two ending in long-term sustainability. These examples indicate that only a joint venture created within the marriage context is sustainable over time.

MARRIAGE PARTNERSHIPS

The Marriage: Party A and Party B
Higher Education Pipelines Case Study

In 2008, I was the president of Congreso de Latinos Unidos, one of the largest Latino human service nonprofit agencies in the country. After an intense Eisenhower Fellowship experience learning from global leaders, I came to understand that to help move people out of poverty, we needed to create higher education opportunities that gave people the tools and credentials to reenter the workforce with employment that could support their families and restore the dignity they lost when they became dependent on government services. Understanding this reality, I sought out David Castro, a fellow Eisenhower and Ashoka Fellow, who had developed a concept and a legal revenue share agreement with a local associate's degree college that allowed this vision to become a reality. Following the analysis, I outline the mutual benefits, motivations, and trust that were in place before both organizations entered into the joint venture.

Benefits

- Breaking the cycle of poverty for low-income populations
- A financially sustainable model (independent of government contracts and grants) for both parties

Motivation

- David Castro was motivated by social impact goals based on his history of social justice work.
- David was also motivated by the prospect of preparing a reasonable number of enrolled students to ensure autonomy in a constantly shifting social sector.

Trust

- I could trust David.
- We were not aware of the trust levels between our respective boards and/or the successors of our organizations regarding honoring the partnership if one of us departed.

Based on the assumption that eventually one organization will in a joint venture attempt to gain financial or governance control over the venture, David and I determined that we needed to enter into a marriage type of partnership in which neither party could exit or change the arrangement without the other's consent. It was understood that Party B owned the legal and financial agreement with the associate's degree college and that Party A owned the building needed to house the program and had the relationship with students. As such, we created a separate for-profit entity that was equally owned by our respective nonprofits with a clearly defined financial agreement. Appendix A is the template of the legal arrangement.

On my departure, the joint venture survived despite being tested both financially and legally by the organizations' boards and successors. A new financial arrangement was agreed upon with the consent of both parties.

The Marriage: Public Health Management Corporation and Congreso de Latinos Unidos

In 2010, I, the president of Congreso de Latinos Unidos (Congreso), was approached by Public Health Management Corporation (PHMC) regarding joining efforts to open a new federally qualified health center (FQHC) in our target area. Congreso had historically been providing preventive health care to the community in an attempt to reduce the high percentage of individuals with diabetes, asthma, heart disease, and other chronic diseases and other health disparities common to minority and very low-income populations. Despite its broad range of services, Congreso was not a primary care provider and thus could not tap into health insurance dollars and other financial benefits available to FQHCs. Congreso's health services were reliant on philanthropic dollars with limited options for growth and sustainability. An FQHC would allow Congreso direct access to health care dollars to serve our people comprehensively and holistically and to ultimately improve their health outcomes. PHMC would be allowed to serve a new market, one considered impossible to enter without preestablished trust relationships, and to help a new population achieve better health outcomes. Following the analysis, I outline the mutual benefits, motivations, and trust that were in place before both organizations entered into the joint venture.

Benefits

- Creating healthy habits and good health in a low-income population

- Managing chronic disease using a holistic, and less expensive, model with a population that did not lend itself to healthy behaviors
- A model that would be financially sustainable (with independent contracts and grants) for both parties

Motivation

- PHMC's motivation was to enter into new markets.

Trust

- I trusted Tine Hansen-Turton, chief strategy officer at PHMC and chief executive officer (CEO) of the National Nursing Centers Consortium, a PHMC affiliate.
- We were not aware of the trust levels between our respective organizations' boards or of any potential successors in terms of honoring the partnership if one of us departed. However, continued support seemed unlikely because both organizations had a history of being the leader within their respective industries.

Given the knowledge of each organization's history, the goal was to set up the partnership such that if either party wanted to walk away, each would walk away with what they brought to the partnership. It was acknowledged that PHMC owned the technical knowledge and experience of operating primary health clinics and had vital relationships with third-party payers, had the grant-writing technical knowledge to apply to be an FQHC, and had the necessary relationship with the federal government. It was acknowledged that Congreso had the trust of the community—thousands of prospective clients—because they had already been serving these clients with their other services. Congreso also had the ideal space where the FQHC could be housed, and the community presence to overcome local politics. Importantly for PHMC, Congreso's existing population of more than 15,000 clients provided an ideal pool from which to solicit survey and surveillance data, as well as qualitative input, all of which informed the assessment of the need for and design of the health center.

Based on the assumption that eventually one organization will attempt to gain financial or governance control over the joint venture, we determined that we needed to enter into a marriage type of partnership in which neither party could exit or change the arrangement without the other's consent. As such, we created a memorandum of agreement (a sample agreement is presented in Chapter 10) that clearly outlined each organization's role, authority, and financial rewards and risks. The agreement was mutually enacted, and then it became our responsibility to sell it to our respective boards. Such an agreement, with each partner having equal "skin in the game" financially, was unique to the health center world. Typically, a partner such as Congreso would simply serve as host/landlord and receive a set fee for rent, facilities, and so on. In this case, in which potential profit was reinvested and potential shortfalls were covered equally, each organization was responsible for ensuring the success of the joint venture. This was particularly appropriate for a fee-for-service-driven industry such as health care, in which the financial bottom line is highly dependent on the design of the workflow and of the physical space in which services will be delivered. For example, if the physical layout of the site or its facilities were not optimal, the host partner, in this case Congreso, would be incentivized to work with PHMC to resolve the problem.

In part due to the financial pressures of the health care industry outlined, primary health care and social services/health promotion organizational cultures are very different. The process of aligning the cultures of each of these large, well-established organizations was a slow one, and trust had to be cultivated among new staff at multiple levels (executive, operations, front line).

On my departure, the joint venture survived despite being tested financially and legally by the organization boards and successors. A new financial and legal arrangement was negotiated and agreed upon with the consent of both parties.

PARENT/CHILD PARTNERSHIPS

Big Picture Philadelphia and Congreso de Latinos Unidos

In 2007, just a few years after returning to Philadelphia and on the heels of working in the national Big Picture Learning Network as a high school cofounder and national network coach, David Bromley was presented with the opportunity of starting a nonprofit Big Picture franchise. His mission was and remains to provide transformative educational opportunities aligned with Big Picture's educational design for Philadelphia's youth.

Big Picture Philadelphia's first opportunity to start a new school came with the release of a request for proposals from the School District of Philadelphia (SDP) seeking organizations interested in establishing alternative schools for overaged but under-credited youth. In the year prior to submitting our proposal, as the executive director of Big Picture Philadelphia, Mr. Bromley had the privilege of meeting with dozens of Philadelphia's more experienced educators and nonprofit leaders. An alternative high school provided him with the chance to reach out and explore potential partnerships with some of these individuals and organizations. In particular, his design team recognized the need to secure a partnership with a strong social services organization to strengthen their proposal and, more importantly, to provide psychological and behavioral wraparound services to the youth they were hoping to serve.

I was one of the first individuals he reached out to, as the president of Congreso de Latinos Unidos (Congreso). During our initial meeting, Mr. Bromley was struck by my passion for education and my belief that the best social services organization was only going to be as effective as the quality of the schools that served its clients. Under my leadership, Congreso supported the founding of Pan America Charter School for K-8 youth and provided local middle and high schools with after-school and on-site behavioral health resources, proving that my belief in developing strong educational partnerships and investing Congreso's time and resources were not just lip service—I was also genuinely enthusiastic about Big Picture's educational design. After Mr. Bromley and I agreed to move forward together to submit a proposal, I offered to convene a meeting during which I introduced him to my leadership team and offered our organization's support.

The first significant partnership choice to be made was which organization would submit the proposal and, if it was approved. would hold the contract with the district. Despite the fact that Big

Picture Philadelphia was a new organization with few resources, Mr. Bromley's board was emphatic about their leading the effort. And as he and I looked more closely at the proposal, it was also clear that 90% of the proposed design, start-up, and support work would be led by Big Picture Philadelphia. Nonetheless, Congreso has many more resources and a strong connection to the eastern north Philadelphia community. In the end, because the proposed work was primarily an education endeavor and because of Big Picture Learning Network's positive reputation, we agreed that Congreso would play a supportive role and Big Picture would submit the proposal.

As the proposal was being developed, Congreso and Big Picture Philadelphia were forced to address legal and financial issues. A name was agreed upon, El Centro de Estudiantes, which represented both the Big Picture philosophy of one student at a time and the Latino clientele that Congreso served. The subheading, "A Big Picture Philadelphia—Congreso School" was also agreed upon. The two parties proposed the development of a school leadership council (SLC) comprising equal membership from both organizations. The SLC would review school data, finances, and staffing.

Specific roles and responsibilities around the operation of the proposed school were also laid out in the proposal, as were the minimum financial commitments from both parties in the form of in-kind services.

A strong working relationship was formed through developing and presenting the proposal. The majority of the proposal was written by Big Picture Philadelphia, while the Congreso leadership and development staff provided editing and solicited letters of support.

On receiving the contract from SDP, the two organizations again worked closely together to open El Centro. Congreso provided the Big Picture Philadelphia leadership team with office space, technology support, and assistance in identifying a facility. Big Picture staff led the hiring effort, staff professional development, and curriculum development. Both organizations worked tirelessly on student recruitment.

El Centro opened in September 2009, and soon some of the proposed collaborative efforts gave way to the tyranny of the immediate that is often associated with opening a school. Unfortunately, as a result, the

SLC never formally developed. Mr. Bromley and I continued to stay in touch, and occasionally we held meetings with representatives from each organization.

The most difficult aspect of the working relationship stemmed from the suddenly very apparent different working patterns of the two organizations. Congreso, being a well-established organization, had expectations of collecting data on all of the clients who fell under their umbrella, including El Centro. The Big Picture Philadelphia staff were more consumed with the day-to-day needs of the staff and students, and they failed to follow through on Congreso's needs. Conversely, the El Centro staff, initially overwhelmed by the trauma-induced behaviors of many of the students, badly wanted daily on-site counseling services to assist with student and family needs. Congreso's staff was unable to provide the on-site person power in part out of frustration with El Centro's inability to help define an ideal caseload size. Nonetheless, until my departure from Congreso toward the end of the second year of El Centro's operations, the two agencies continued to try and redefine the relationship and how Congreso could provide behavioral support.

Here I outline the benefits, motivation, and trust that were in place before either organization entered into this joint venture.

Benefits

- Creating an alternative option for young people who had dropped out of high school.
- The model would be financially sustainable because it was contracted by the School District of Philadelphia.

Motivation

- Big Picture's motivation was to serve students who were not successful in the traditional high school model.
- Congreso's motivation was to offer lasting and sustainable impact in the form of high school diplomas for the young people they served every day.

Trust

- Mr. Bromley and I trusted each other in the sense that we were willing to work together to achieve the agreed-upon social impact goals.
- We were not aware of the trust levels between our respective organizations' boards and/or successors in terms of honoring a partnership if one of us departed. Understanding that one organization had to be the lead applicant, both parties agreed that Big Picture Philadelphia was the organization that had the education expertise.

On my departure, the relationship between the organizations completely changed with the arrival of Congreso's new executive director, who believed that since there was nothing to be gained financially by the Big Picture relationship, it made no sense for Congreso to continue to spend time and energy on the endeavor. Simply stated, a business decision was made over a social impact decision. Ultimately, Big Picture kept the school and raised enough private funds to develop a counseling team that provides on-site counseling and makes referrals to behavioral support agencies across North Philadelphia, including Congreso.

The upshot is that only joint ventures framed within a marriage context have the ability to withstand time and become sustainable. Joint ventures are difficult, and unless they are legally and/or financially binding, it is too easy for either party to walk away and not do the hard work required for the venture. Interestingly, on a side note, the individuals who originated these partnerships continue to work together to create new partnerships, whereas only 50% of the actual organization joint ventures continued.

APPENDIX A: LIMITED LIABILITY COMPANY OPERATING AGREEMENT

A Member-Managed Limited Liability Company

THIS OPERATING AGREEMENT is made and entered into effective July 1, 2009, by and among: Party A ("Party A") and Party B, Inc. ("Party B") (collectively referred to in this agreement as the "Members").

SECTION 1

The Limited Liability Company

1.1 Formation. Effective July 1, 2009, the Members form a limited liability company under the name ORGANIZATION NAME (the "Company") on the terms and conditions in this Operating Agreement (the "Agreement") and pursuant to the Pennsylvania Limited Liability Company Law of 1994 (the "Act"). The Members agree to file with the appropriate agency within the Commonwealth of Pennsylvania charged with processing and maintaining such records all documentation required for the formation of the Company. The rights and obligations of the parties are as provided in the Act, except as otherwise expressly provided in this Agreement.

1.2 Name. The business of the Company will be conducted under the name ORGANIZATION NAME, LLC, or such other name upon which the Members may unanimously agree.

1.3 Purpose. The purpose of the Company is to engage in any lawful act or activity that a Limited Liability Company may carry out under the Act; provided, however, that the Company does not engage in any activity that would threaten the tax-exempt status of any Member that is a tax-exempt organization under Section 501(c)(3) of the Internal Revenue Code of 1986, as amended (the "Code").

1.4 Office. The Company will maintain its principal business office within the Commonwealth of Pennsylvania at the following address: _____. The Members may from time to time change the principal business office and establish additional offices.

1.5 Registered Agent. Party A will serve as the Company's initial registered agent in the Commonwealth of Pennsylvania, and the registered office is _____.

1.6 Term. The term of the Company commences on the date of its registration with the Commonwealth of Pennsylvania and shall continue perpetually unless sooner terminated as provided in this Agreement.

1.7 Names and Addresses of Members. The Members' names and addresses are attached as Schedule 1 to this Agreement.

1.8 Admission of Additional Members. Except as otherwise expressly provided in this Agreement, no additional members may be admitted to the Company through issuance by the company of a new interest in the Company without the prior unanimous written consent of the Members.

SECTION 2

Capital Contributions

2.1 Initial Contributions. The Members initially shall contribute to the Company capital as described in Schedule 2 attached to this Agreement.

2.2 Additional Contributions. No Member shall be obligated to make any additional contribution to the Company's capital without the prior unanimous written consent of the Members.

2.3 No Interest on Capital Contributions. Members are not entitled to interest or other compensation for or on account of their capital contributions to the Company except to the extent, if any, expressly provided in this Agreement.

SECTION 3

Allocation of Profits and Losses; Distributions

3.1 Profits and Losses. For financial accounting and tax purposes, the Company's net profits and net losses shall be determined annually and allocated to the Members in proportion to each Member's relative ownership interest in the Company as set forth in Schedule 2, as may be amended from time to time, and in accordance with U.S. Department of the Treasury Regulation 1.704–1.

3.2 Distributions. The Members shall determine and distribute available funds annually or at more frequent intervals as they see fit. Available funds, as referred to herein, shall mean the net cash of the Company available after appropriate provision for expenses and liabilities, as determined by the Members. Distributions in liquidation of the Company or in liquidation of a Member's interest shall be made in accordance with positive capital account balances pursuant to U.S. Department of the Treasury Regulation 1.704.1(b)(2)(ii)(b)(2). When a Member has a negative capital account balance, there shall be a qualified income offset, as set forth in U.S. Department of the Treasury Regulation 1.704.1(b)(2)(ii)(d).

3.3 No Right to Demand Return of Capital. No Member has any right to any return of capital or other distribution except as expressly provided in this Agreement. No Member has any drawing account with the Company.

SECTION 4

Indemnification

The Company shall indemnify any person who was or is a party defendant or is threatened to be made a party defendant, to any pending or completed action, suit, or proceeding, whether civil, criminal, administrative, or investigative (other than an action by or in the right of the Company) because of being a member, manager, employee or agent of the Company, or is or was serving at the request of the Company, against expenses (including attorney's fees), judgments, fines, and amounts paid in settlement actually and reasonably incurred in connection with such action, suit, or proceeding if the Members determine that the employee acted in good faith and in a manner reasonably believed to be in or not opposed to the best interest of the Company, and that with respect to any criminal action proceeding, they have no reasonable cause to believe the employee's conduct was unlawful, provided, however, that the Company shall not indemnify, defend, or hold harmless any Member who violates such lesser standard of conduct or public policy for which applicable law or Sections 501(c)(3) or 4958 of the Code would prevent or not permit indemnification hereunder. The termination of any action, suit, or proceeding by judgment, order, settlement, or conviction or upon a plea of "no lo contendere" or its equivalent shall not in itself create a presumption that the person did or did not act in good faith and in a manner that he reasonably believed to be in the best interest of the Company, and, with respect to any criminal action or proceeding, had reasonable cause to believe that his/her conduct was lawful.

SECTION 5

Powers and Duties of Managers

5.1 Management of Company.

    5.1.1 The Members, within the authority granted by the Act and the terms of this Agreement shall have the complete power and authority to manage and operate the Company and make all decisions affecting its business and affairs.

    5.1.2 Except as otherwise provided in this Agreement, all decisions and documents relating to the management and operation of the Company shall be made and executed by a Majority in Interest of the Members.

    5.1.3 Third parties dealing with the Company shall be entitled to rely conclusively upon the power and authority of a Majority in Interest of the Members to manage and operate the business and affairs of the Company.

5.2 Decisions by Members. Whenever in this Agreement reference is made to the decision, consent, approval, judgment, or action of the

Members, unless otherwise expressly provided in this Agreement, such decision, consent, approval, judgment, or action shall mean a Majority of the Members.

5.3 Withdrawal by a Member. A Member has no power to withdraw from the Company, except as otherwise provided in Section 8.

SECTION 6

Salaries, Reimbursement, and Payment of Expenses

6.1 Organization Expenses. All expenses incurred in connection with organization of the Company will be paid by the Company.

6.2 Salary. No salary will be paid to a Member for the performance of his or her duties under this Agreement unless the salary has been approved in writing by a Majority of the Members.

6.3 Legal and Accounting Services. The Company may obtain legal and accounting services to the extent reasonably necessary for the conduct of the Company's business.

SECTION 7

Books of Account, Accounting Reports, Tax Returns, Fiscal Year, Banking

7.1 Method of Accounting. The Company will use the method of accounting previously determined by the Members for financial reporting and tax purposes.

7.2 Fiscal Year; Taxable Year. The fiscal year and the taxable year of the Company is July 1 to June 30.

7.3 Capital Accounts. The Company will maintain a Capital Account for each Member on a cumulative basis in accordance with federal income tax accounting principles.

7.4 Banking. All funds of the Company will be deposited in a separate bank account or in an account or accounts of a savings and loan association in the name of the Company as determined by a Majority of the Members. Company funds will be invested or deposited with an institution, the accounts or deposits of which are insured or guaranteed by an agency of the United States government.

SECTION 8

Transfer of Membership Interest

8.1 Sale or Encumbrance Prohibited. Except as otherwise permitted in this Agreement, no Member may voluntarily or involuntarily transfer, sell, convey, encumber, pledge, assign, or otherwise dispose of (collectively, "Transfer") an interest in the Company without the prior written consent of a majority of the other nontransferring Members determined on a per capita basis.

8.2 Right of First Refusal. Notwithstanding Section 8.1, a Member may transfer all or any part of the Member's interest in the Company (the "Interest") as follows:

8.2.1 The Member desiring to transfer his or her Interest first must provide written notice (the "Notice") to the other Members, specifying the price and terms on which the Member is prepared to sell the Interest (the "Offer").

8.2.2 For a period of 30 days after receipt of the Notice, the Members may acquire all, but not less than all, of the Interest at the price and under the terms specified in the Offer. If the other Members desiring to acquire the Interest cannot agree among themselves on the allocation of the Interest among them, the allocation will be proportional to the Ownership Interests of those Members desiring to acquire the Interest.

8.2.3 Closing of the sale of the Interest will occur as stated in the Offer; provided, however, that the closing will not be less than 45 days after expiration of the 30-day notice period.

8.2.4 If the other Members fail or refuse to notify the transferring Member of their desire to acquire all of the Interest proposed to be transferred within the 30-day period following receipt of the Notice, then the Members will be deemed to have waived their right to acquire the Interest on the terms described in the Offer, and the transferring Member may sell and convey the Interest consistent with the Offer to any other person or entity; provided, however, that notwithstanding anything in Section 8.2 to the contrary, should the sale to a third person be at a price or on terms that are more favorable to the purchaser than stated in the Offer, then the transferring Member must reoffer the sale of the Interest to the remaining Members at that other price or other terms; provided, further, that if the sale to a third person is not closed within 6 months after the expiration of the 30-day period described above, then the provisions of Section 8.2 will again apply to the Interest proposed to be sold or conveyed.

8.3 Substituted Parties. Any transfer in which the Transferee becomes a fully substituted Member is not permitted unless and until:

(1) The transferor and assignee execute and deliver to the Company the documents and instruments of conveyance necessary or appropriate in the opinion of counsel to the Company to effect the transfer and to confirm the agreement of the permitted assignee to be bound by the provisions of this Agreement; and

(2) The transferor furnishes to the Company an opinion of counsel, satisfactory to the Company, that the transfer will not cause the Company to terminate for federal income tax purposes or that any termination is not adverse to the Company or the other Members.

8.4 Dissolution, or Bankruptcy of Member. On the dissolution or bankruptcy of a Member, unless the Company exercises its rights under Section 8.5, the successor in interest to the Member (whether an estate, bankruptcy trustee, or otherwise) will receive only the economic right to receive distributions whenever made by the Company and the Member's allocable share of taxable income, gain, loss, deduction, and credit (the "Economic Rights") unless and until a majority of the other Members determined on a per capita basis admit the transferee as a fully substituted Member in accordance with the provisions of Section 8.3.

8.4.1 Any transfer of Economic Rights pursuant to Section 8.4 will not include any right to participate in management of the Company, including any right to vote, consent to, and will not include any right to information on the Company or its operations or financial condition. Following any transfer of only the Economic Rights of a Member's Interest in the Company, the transferring Member's power and right to vote or consent to any matter submitted to the Members will be eliminated, and the Ownership Interests of the remaining Members, for purposes only of such votes, consents, and participation in management, will be proportionately increased until such time, if any, as the transferee of the Economic Rights becomes a fully substituted Member.

SECTION 9

Dissolution and Winding Up of the Company

9.1 Dissolution. The Company will be dissolved on the happening of any of the following events:

9.1.1 Sale, transfer, or other disposition of all or substantially all of the property of the Company;

9.1.2 The agreement of all of the Members;

9.1.3 By operation of law; or

9.1.4 The dissolution, or bankruptcy of a Member or the revocation of the tax-exempt status of a Member, as an organization described in Section 501(c)(3) of the Code, or the occurrence of any event that terminates the continued membership of a Member in the Company, unless there are then remaining at least the minimum number of Members required by law and all of the remaining Members, within 120 days after the date of the event, elect to continue the business of the Company.

9.2 Winding Up. On the dissolution of the Company (if the Company is not continued), the Members must take full account of the Company's assets and liabilities, and the assets will be liquidated as promptly as is consistent with obtaining their fair value, and the proceeds, to the extent sufficient to pay the Company's obligations with respect to the liquidation, will be applied and distributed, after any gain or loss realized in connection with the liquidation has been allocated in accordance with Section 3 of this Agreement, and the Members' Capital Accounts have been adjusted to reflect the allocation and all other transactions through the date of the distribution, in the following order:

9.2.1 To payment and discharge of the expenses of liquidation and of all the Company's debts and liabilities to persons or organizations other than Members;

9.2.2 To the payment and discharge of any Company debts and liabilities owed to Members; and

9.2.3 To Members in the amount of their respective adjusted Capital Account balances on the date of distribution; provided, however, that any then-outstanding Default Advances (with interest and costs of collection) first must be repaid from distributions otherwise allocable to the Defaulting Member pursuant to Section 9.2.3.

SECTION 10

General Provisions

10.1 Amendments. Amendments to this Agreement may be proposed by any Member. A proposed amendment will be adopted and become effective as an amendment only on the written approval of all of the Members.

10.2 Governing Law. This Agreement and the rights and obligations of the parties under it are governed by and interpreted in accordance with the laws of the Commonwealth of Pennsylvania (without regard to principles of conflicts of law).

10.3 Entire Agreement; Modification. This Agreement constitutes the entire understanding and agreement between the Members with respect to the subject matter of this Agreement. No agreements, understandings, restrictions, representations, or warranties exist between or among the members other than those in this Agreement or referred to or provided for in this Agreement. No modification or amendment of any provision of this Agreement will be binding on any Member unless in writing and signed by all the Members.

10.4 Attorney Fees. In the event of any suit or action to enforce or interpret any provision of this Agreement (or that is based on this

Agreement), the prevailing party is entitled to recover, in addition to other costs, reasonable attorney fees in connection with the suit, action, or arbitration, and in any appeals. The determination of who is the prevailing Party and the amount of reasonable attorney fees to be paid to the prevailing party will be decided by the court or courts, including any appellate courts, in which the matter is tried, heard, or decided.

10.5 Further Effect. The parties agree to execute other documents reasonably necessary to further effect and evidence the terms of this Agreement, as long as the terms and provisions of the other documents are fully consistent with the terms of this Agreement.

10.6 Severability. If any term or provision of this Agreement is held to be void or unenforceable, that term or provision will be severed from this Agreement, the balance of the Agreement will survive, and the balance of this Agreement will be reasonably construed to carry out the intent of the parties as evidenced by the terms of this Agreement.

10.7 Captions. The captions used in this Agreement are for the convenience of the parties only and will not be interpreted to enlarge, contract, or alter the terms and provisions of this Agreement.

10.8 Notices. All notices required to be given by this Agreement will be in writing and will be effective when actually delivered or, if mailed, when deposited as certified mail, postage prepaid, directed to the addresses first shown above for each Member or to such other address as a Member may specify by notice given in conformance with these provisions to the other Members.

IN WITNESS WHEREOF, the parties to this Agreement execute this Operating Agreement as of the date and year first above written.

Members

Party A.

BY: _____

President and CEO

Party B, Inc.

BY: _____

President and CEO

Listing of Members - Schedule 1

LIMITED LIABILITY COMPANY OPERATING AGREEMENT
FOR ORGANIZATION NAME, LLC

Listing of Members

As of the 1st day of _____, the following is a list of Members of the Company:

1. Party A.
   ADDRESS

2. Party B.
   ADDRESS

Authorized by Member(s) to provide Member Listing as of this 1st day of _____.

Party A.

BY: _____

President and CEO

Party B, Inc.

BY: _____

President and CEO

Listing of Capital Contributions - Schedule 2

LIMITED LIABILITY COMPANY OPERATING AGREEMENT
FOR ORGANIZATION NAME, LLC

Capital Contributions

Pursuant to ARTICLE 2, each Member's initial contribution to the Company capital is stated to be $1,000. The description and each individual portion of this initial contribution are as follows:

NAME:	Party A	Party B
CONTRIBUTION:	$1,000	$1,000
OWNERSHIP:	50%	50%

SIGNED AND AGREED as of this 1st day of _____.

Party A.

BY: _____

President and CEO

Party B, Inc.

BY: _____

President and CEO

LIMITED LIABILITY COMPANY OPERATING AGREEMENT
FOR ORGANIZATION NAME, LLC

Valuation of Member Interest

Pursuant to ARTICLE 8, the initial value of each Member's interest in the Company is endorsed as follows:

NAME:	VALUATION	ENDORSEMENT
Party A:	$1,000	
Party B:	$1,000	

SIGNED AND AGREED as of this 1st day of _____.

Party A.

BY: _____

President and CEO

Party B, Inc.

BY: _____

President and CEO

7

Administrative Consolidations, Administrative Services Organizations, and Joint Programming

Nicholas D. Torres, Jacob Cavallo, Arun Prabhakaran, and Tivoni Devor

EDITORS' OVERVIEW

Thomas McLaughlin briefly discussed administrative partnerships back in Chapter 3. This chapter features a series of case studies and best practices for partnerships that discuss in detail the provision of back-office support for nonprofit partners.

Nonprofit organizations, such as management corporations that offer back-office support, usually provide financially and operationally feasible solutions. Public Health Management Corporation (PHMC) is a nonprofit public health institute that creates and sustains healthier communities using best practices to improve community health through direct service, partnership, innovation, policy, research, technical assistance, and a prepared work force. PHMC, headquartered in Philadelphia, operates as a management company and has served greater Philadelphia since 1972. Since 2000, the company and its affiliate partners have served Pennsylvania, Delaware, and southern New

Jersey, and it reaches all 50 states and the District of Columbia through affiliate partners. PHMC fulfills its mission to improve community health by providing back-office support services, outreach, health promotion, education, research, planning, technical assistance, and direct services to nonprofits and government. PHMC has 12 affiliates, of which 3 are support affiliates.

Traditional back-office services are usually designed to address many of the challenges of today's changing nonprofit environment. From improving communications with funders and donors to solving mission-critical initiatives and increasing human resource and operating efficiencies, technical and management service offerings bring practical, strategic, proactive consulting services and products that are tailored to meet the needs of client organizations.

Services depend on the level of organizational need and affordability, but are usually identified through a comprehensive organizational assessment of the nonprofit client. These services usually include:

- Human resources (HR)
  - HR outsourcing and consulting services, including payroll and tax administration, workers' compensation, unemployment, compliance, and benefits administration, including health, life, dental, and disability insurance, voluntary benefits, executive benefits, health and wellness benefits consulting services, and retirement plan services
  - Risk management services in professional employer organizations
  - Flexible end-to-end payroll services for companies
  - Co-employment relationships with client companies
  - A complete HR solution, including all aspects of payroll, compliance, risk management, and employee benefit procurement and administration
  - Commercial insurance policies
- Finance and accounting
  - Analyzing client organizations' operations, determining financially and operationally feasible solutions, and helping to ensure the successful implementation of those solutions
  - Assisting with improving communications with funders and donors to solve mission-critical initiatives and increase operating efficiencies

- ○ Devising technical and management consulting service offerings that bring practical, strategic, proactive services and products that are tailored to meet the needs of client organizations
- ○ Based on need, fiscal management support (FMS) can include serving as the organization's chief financial officer, controller, accountant, and bookkeeper (FMS helps organizations implement procedures that ensure greater control, transparency, and compliance with federal, state, and local reporting requirements)
- ○ Accounts receivable (mailing out invoices, tracking revenue, posting sales figures)
- ○ Accounts payable (posting vendor invoices, posting and printing checks, tracking credit invoices, vendor payments)
- ○ Month-end transactions and financial statements (reconciling bank statements, monthly journal entries, and income statements with monthly and year-to-date figures, balance sheets, profit & loss statements, etc.)
- ○ Year-end documentation (preparation of books for accountant at year-end to assist in filing tax returns, W-2 preparation and reconciliation, closing out fiscal year accounts, profit & loss statements, etc.)
- ○ Assessments, benchmarking, budgeting and forecasting, evaluations, troubleshooting
- ○ Financial analysis and reporting, including cash flow issues
- ○ Fiscal responsibility training for board members and other staff
- ○ Internal controls
- • Program development and fundraising
  - ○ Fiscal sponsorship
  - ○ Proposal development in response to requests for proposals and other funding opportunities
  - ○ Fundraising strategies and assistance
  - ○ Grant management and administration
  - ○ Program development and guidance
- • Quality assurance
  - ○ Total quality management (quality assurance integration and management support)

- o Training and corporate compliance assistance
- o Health Insurance Portability and Accountability Act and other privacy adherence
- o Standards of care
- o Privacy and confidentiality consultation
- o Regulatory compliance
- Marketing and communications
  - o Broad-based marketing and internal and external communications support
  - o Messaging, branding, and design support
- Information technology (IT)
  - o Centralized IT solutions (maintaining computers, networks, and other IT services)
  - o IT support and technical assistance
  - o Help desk support (if integrated)
  - o Database management
  - o IT customization
  - o Programming
- Executive management and administration
  - o Corporate-wide strategy support for senior management and leadership
  - o Government and community relations and strategic support
  - o Business and strategic planning
  - o Business process reengineering
  - o Strategic partnerships, joint ventures, mergers, and affiliations

---

FISCAL SPONSORSHIP: THE URBAN AFFAIRS COALITION MODEL

Jacob Cavallo and Arun Prabhakaran

INTRODUCTION

- The Urban Affairs Coalition (UAC) is a Philadelphia-based nonprofit that was founded in 1969 following a historic meeting between the city's business and community leaders. For more than 45 years, UAC has united government, business, neighborhood, and individual initiatives to improve the quality of life in the region and solve emerging issues.

- In 1969, a historic partnership between business and community leaders was formed, creating The Philadelphia Urban Coalition. Nicknamed "The Urb," its purpose was to eliminate poverty, discrimination, and civic unrest and to secure human and civil rights. Through the 1980s, alliances grew with the founding of The Urban Affairs Partnership, an organization created to improve the quality of life in greater Philadelphia. In 1991, The Urban Affairs Partnership and the Philadelphia Urban Coalition merged to create the Greater Philadelphia Urban Affairs Coalition. In early 2010, the Greater Philadelphia Urban Affairs Coalition shed "Greater Philadelphia" from its name to acknowledge the opportunities for growth and services in the full five-county region and beyond.

- Since its formation, UAC has carved out a niche as a "home for nonprofits." In this capacity, UAC supports more than 55 programs and 15 projects, including a host of nationally recognized initiatives (www.uac.org/partners-programs). UAC provides nonprofits with core services that help them remain high impact and cost efficient. By adopting UAC's model of fiscal sponsorship and shared services, nonprofits are equipped with the essential tools they need to thrive while reducing their overhead. This has had a direct and immediate benefit for the people these nonprofits serve.

- UAC's fiscal sponsorship offering grew organically out of its role as a community problem solver in Philadelphia, through which it found that many organizations struggled with the compliance and administration requirements of government contracts. The Coalition saw this challenge as an opportunity to leverage its experience with managing government funds, which became a formalized service offering to other organizations. The value of this service grew along with the trend of the increased outsourcing of government services to the growing nonprofit sector in the 1980s and 1990s.

A BRIEF LOOK AT FISCAL SPONSORSHIP

- Fiscal sponsorship is a formal legal arrangement in which a 501(c)(3) public charity sponsors a group or project, allowing it to share the sponsor's legal and tax-exempt status. The sponsored organization shares with its sponsors a similar mission and set of goals. Organizations elect fiscal sponsorship because of the cost-saving and shared-service benefits that often result from this partnership.
- Fiscal sponsorship arrangements generally occur between established nonprofits and smaller organizations that want to have access to the infrastructure and tax-related benefits that a large organization can provide. As a result, the sponsoring organization will provide consulting, oversight in the form of feedback, and in-house administrative services, some or all of which can be used by the sponsored organization.
- Because fiscal sponsorship arrangements confer shared legal and tax statuses, the sponsoring organization assumes a degree of responsibility for the outcomes of those nonprofits it sponsors. The level of responsibility depends on the needs of the sponsored organization and the terms of the sponsorship arrangement. This can range from complete fiduciary responsibility to providing the oversight necessary to satisfy the Internal Revenue Service (IRS) that the sponsored organization is fulfilling its charitable purpose requirements.
- The ultimate goal of fiscal sponsorship varies based on the needs of the sponsored organization. Nonprofits come in all shapes and sizes, and their needs are equally diverse. The nonprofits that take advantage of fiscal sponsorship do so because they stand to benefit from the arrangement.
- Often, people interested in starting a nonprofit begin by trying to obtain 501(c)(3) status from the IRS. However, this process is expensive and time-consuming: It can take up to a year and cost several thousand dollars to gain approval for an application. In addition, there are filings for local incorporation documents and the time needed to assemble all of the various related documentation, which often exceeds 100 pages of material (Woodward, 2013).

In contrast, an organization might in as few as 30 days (based on the time it takes for a typical organization to become sponsored by UAC) find a fiscal sponsor so that they can share the sponsoring organization's 501(c)(3) status. This allows them to immediately receive tax-deductible donations and apply for grants that require tax-exempt status.

Types of Fiscal Sponsorship and Other Services Offered by UAC

- UAC has equipped itself with the tools necessary to assist non-profits, mostly grassroots organizations with revenues of less than $5 million. While there are a number of sponsorship models, most of UAC's arrangements involve comprehensive fiscal sponsorship. UAC also provides preapproved grant relationship and technical assistance sponsorship models.

Comprehensive Fiscal Sponsorship

- Comprehensive fiscal sponsorship (also referred to as Model A fiscal sponsorship; fiscal sponsorship models are taken from Colvin, 2006a) occurs when a fiscal sponsor provides an organization with all of its administrative needs. This model is often used by small- to medium-sized organizations, especially newly forming organizations. The fiscal sponsor manages finance and accounting, payroll, hiring, HR, and benefits. The sponsor also generally provides a large degree of support to its sponsored program. In most cases, the sponsored program has access to all of its sponsor's resources.
- While the sponsored program retains its autonomy, it becomes no different in a legal sense than any other activity that the sponsor would carry out. The sponsor has full liability for the actions of the program and its employees. Therefore, it is customary for a sponsor and its member organizations to have detailed sponsorship agreements, often in the form of a memorandum of understanding, that describe the terms and conditions of the relationship. For

example, both organizations must agree beforehand what will occur in the event that a project decides to become its own legal entity or if a project fulfills its goal and decides to cease activity.

- For new organizations, fiscal sponsorship offers them "speed to market," with immediate access to all of the benefits that come from large organizations without any of the costs. They do not need to invest in the infrastructure for dedicated HR, accounting, and IT departments; they have total access to the skilled professionals of the parent organization whenever they need them.

- Comprehensive fiscal sponsorship is also the main choice for new initiatives or partnerships that form as the result of public–private collaborations. These projects do not need to secure office space or incorporate before they can have an impact. Neighborhood organizations, such as community development corporations, can apply for fiscal sponsorship, and, once they meet the sponsoring organization's requirements, they can immediately begin fundraising and program activities. They do not need to undergo the lengthy process of attaining IRS charitable status before they begin operating. These organizations choose fiscal sponsorship because of the tax exemption they receive when they are sponsored.

- The comprehensive fiscal sponsorship model is the least exposed to legal or IRS challenges. This method has been called the best training ground for start-up projects (Colvin, 2006a). Because of the immediate and long-term benefits of comprehensive fiscal sponsorship, the majority of organizations that are a part of UAC elect to use this model.

Preapproved Grant Relationship

- Subsets of organizations that apply for fiscal sponsorship (this depends on the sponsorship agreement) conduct their own fundraising and long-term planning while remaining under the umbrella of the sponsoring organization.

- These organizations often apply for grants in the name of their fiscal sponsor. When this happens, the relationship is classified as a preapproved grant relationship (or Model C fiscal sponsorship).

The sponsor provides the project funds only to the extent that money is received from donors.

- Grants and tax-deductible donations can then be made to the sponsor and passed on to the sponsored organization, which is already its own legally incorporated entity. The fiscal sponsor carefully administers funds to make sure that grant dollars are used as proposed by the sponsored organization. Autonomy and liability vary based on the terms set forth in the fiscal sponsorship agreement.

Technical Assistance

- Technical assistance (Model F) is provided on a fee-for-service basis to organizations that wish to maintain their own 501(c)(3) status. Under this relationship, organizations select from a range of services to suit their needs and pay for them on a graduated fee scale based on revenue and services used. In these cases, technical assistance provision is the only relationship between UAC and the sponsored organization.

Other Services

- Beyond these services, UAC provides nonprofits with a range of tailored back-office and shared services, often at a lower price point and with greater quality than other alternatives. By layering these services on top of fiscal sponsorship, UAC has gained an economy of scale and efficiency—and at typically a lower cost—than the sponsored organizations could access through outside firms or retaining functions in-house.
- Reducing risk and overhead through shared services is a prime reason organizations choose to work with UAC; in some cases, they save hundreds of thousands of dollars. Key areas in which organizations save money include employee benefits, insurance coverage, audit expenses, vendor contracts, and other services for which purchasing power can be pooled effectively.
- Not every nonprofit is a shining example of impact and cost efficiency. Some underperform, and one of UAC's most important

roles is its ability to provide tailored consulting. These services include: staff training, strategic planning, embedded executives, situational management, financial advice, cost-control recommendations, and turnaround services.

AN IN-DEPTH LOOK AT THE UAC MODEL

- UAC is one of the few nonprofits in the United States that has provided fiscal sponsorship since before the 1980s. It is an established operator with systems and procedures specifically designed for the purpose of fiscal sponsorship. Its focus on fiscal sponsorship allows it to provide services and harness economies of scale that other fiscal sponsors are unable to do.
- From its origins, UAC has had an emphasis on grassroots community initiatives (the Workforce Investment Act classifies grassroots organizations as those with budgets of $500,000 or below). UAC is composed of upward of 70% grassroots initiatives (UAC, 2010, pp. 3–4) with operating budgets under $500,000.
- These grassroots programs serve to innovate at the community level, helping traditionally hard-to-reach populations such as the homeless, ex-offenders, and people living with HIV/AIDS. UAC focuses on organizations that seek to empower individuals who want to be forces for change in their communities by providing them with all of the support of a highly developed infrastructure.

A Broad Network and a Strong Framework for Strategic Partnerships

- Throughout its history, UAC has established a reputation as a trusted community partner, convener, and connector, with a board composed of experienced corporate and community leaders. Because of its age and size, UAC has a multitude of established contacts within the charitable community. Its knowledge base and network are essential for forming inter-organization partnerships. Nonprofits are able to accomplish more by working together than they can alone.

- In the Philadelphia area, UAC has earned a reputation as a stable and reliable operator and frequently works with corporate and government leaders on community initiatives. These relationships often result in nonprofits' being encouraged to join UAC for its services by their corporate board member or government agencies.
- UAC is one of the best-equipped organizations in the city to form new charitable initiatives. Rather than a program's becoming part of the City of Philadelphia, it becomes a part of UAC. Many of the most impactful programs in the city are the result of nonprofit-government partnerships.

Economies of Scale and Cost Savings

- Generally speaking, organizations that have budgets of more than $5,000,000 can generate the revenue needed to support dedicated internal resources for their own HR, legal, and IT departments. It is typically organizations with budgets less than $5 million that can find ways to slash costs, access talent, and improve impact through collaboration.
- Most nonprofits find benefit in shared-services arrangements (Leach & Management Assistance Group, Inc., 2009). However, few nonprofits have the capability or desire to operate these services, implement them, or own them. By layering shared services on top of fiscal sponsorship, UAC works to maximize the cost savings across the entire pool of organizations, in particular, when dealing with for-profit vendors. For example, UAC is able to provide better insurance and employee benefits at a lower cost than independent nonprofits can find in the market because of its buying power.
- One of the greatest impacts of the UAC model is its ability to save partner nonprofits time and money, which can be reinvested in mission work. Another reason a nonprofit might seek out a fiscal sponsorship arrangement with UAC is that the organization might wish to make use of the shared administrative services that an established operator can provide. Rather than their spending time and money on legal, financial, and HR matters, these tasks can be outsourced to the parent organization, which already has the infrastructure to accomplish them efficiently. According to

one internal study, UAC was able to save its 77 program partners a combined total of $1,150,000 during fiscal year 2009. This translates into real dollars that remain in communities through program expenditures and more effective impact.

- The UAC model is also differentiated by the breadth of services it offers. It is one of only 20% of fiscal sponsors who provide their programs with dedicated HR resources, and one of the 22% that provides IT services and consulting (Green, Kvaternik, Alarcon, & LaFrance Associates, LLC., 2006). As nonprofits become more aware of the benefits of fiscal sponsorship, it is likely that there will be an increase in professionalization and variety in the field. UAC is at the forefront of this trend.

Administrative Benefits

- Overhead is a necessary part of any organization, but not all overhead is equal. Without necessary accounting, record keeping, or maintenance, an organization cannot function. All organizations, whether they are nonprofits, businesses, or even government programs, need to invest in overhead to accomplish their goals. An efficient organization will reduce overhead costs as much as possible while still maintaining best practices and administrative capabilities.
- It may seem contradictory that organizations that most need better back-office services may not gain short-term costs savings from fiscal sponsorship. Jeff Russell, an outsourcing expert, said it best when he wrote, "Nonprofits that are spending very little to perform a function poorly won't save money by transferring it to an outside firm. However, the long-term benefits and cost savings could be significant if outsourcing means the executive director and other key staff can spend more time on program and strategy" (Russell, 2013, p. 73).
- In new or small organizations, many of the back-office and administrative tasks are taken care of by executive directors or other senior staff. As a result, small nonprofits can suffer from inattention or inefficiency related to common business management issues, inexperience, and neglect of back-office functions.

- Human resources needs are an excellent example of this challenge. The industry standard for HR staffing is to have one HR professional per 100 employees. It is not realistic for smaller organizations to hire dedicated HR staff, so HR work typically falls on the executive director or another staff member whose expertise may lie in other matters. This can expose the organization to risk when they need to manage HR matters such as attempting to stay current with legal or regulatory changes, or worse. A single HR lawsuit could damage an organization beyond repair.
- Some nonprofits try to solve this issue by contracting out work to for-profits. While this solution is commonplace, it is not the most efficient. A good fiscal sponsor will work for cost and within the budget of an existing nonprofit. Depending on the services provided, a fiscal sponsor can ask for a percentage of revenue to use as an administrative fee. For smaller organizations, it is much more cost-effective to work through a fiscal sponsor rather than hiring, say, an accounting firm.
- The level of specialization offered by UAC frees up both money and time for the sponsored nonprofits. Executive directors can focus on developing new programs and repurpose overhead savings to program expenses.

Legal Support, Tax Benefits, and Risk Management

- Most independent nonprofits struggle when facing complex problems, and often make costly errors. Organizations tend to rely on pro bono support, like a board member, or to pay an outside firm or consultant to resolve many of these problems.
- Finances are also made more transparent with the UAC model of fiscal sponsorship. One criticism made in the early days of fiscal sponsorship was that the process could act as "mere conduits for the transmission of deductible donations to entities not qualified to receive them" (Colvin, 2006b, p. 2). This is not the case with reputable operators such as UAC. There are incredibly strong internal systems and higher-level talent devoted to the fiscal oversight. Due diligence on financial matters is conducted by UAC staff with oversight from UAC's audit and finance committee, which

comprises a number of seasoned professionals from banking, public finance corporations, and auditing firms.

- UAC's accumulated experience and established systems, which were developed over decades, provide organizations with extensive support on compliance and risk management issues. At its scale, UAC can afford talented staff members—masters of business administration (MBAs), certified public accountants (CPAs), lawyers, and other content matter experts—who are seasoned professionals with expertise in a variety of business-related problems. These resources are readily available for UAC's sponsored organizations, and access to these professionals is an important benefit to groups when it comes to reviewing contracts, maintaining financial and regulatory compliance, managing vendors, and more.

Instant Legitimacy

- For many smaller organizations, joining UAC confers legitimacy to fledgling efforts, increasing funder or donor confidence. After a nonprofit joins UAC, it is often able to raise more funds from its existing donors because the donors recognize the positive organizational changes and long-term growth potential that UAC brings. In one case, this was as much as 10% of the entire budget. For an organization with a budget in millions of dollars, a 10% increase in revenue can make a huge difference.

Shared Space

- UAC uses its offices as a de facto nonprofit center, providing lower-than-market-rate rent to tenants in its seven-story facility. This allows organizations to share resources such as Internet, IT support, photocopying, and other facilities-related expenses. This colocation encourages collaboration between organizations because the groups frequently brainstorm or work together on joint projects that serve the community, including essential services, youth development, job training, and community small-business development.

- UAC leverages fiscal sponsorship as an important tool that newly created nonprofits can take advantage of in order to build their organizations. From inception, these projects have access to UAC's resources and expertise. While they are sponsored, these projects are able to work and grow, gaining valuable experience. In this capacity, UAC provides a pipeline to sustainability. Once a project is established, its leadership may decide to seek independence or continue the relationship with UAC.
- In all of these examples, fiscal sponsorship with the UAC model is chosen because it makes sense for the organization at its stage of development. Sometimes, the reason is as simple as finding cost savings, and at other times, the reason is far more complex; UAC may be able to provide the technical assistance necessary for an organization to thrive. In all cases, both organizations stand to benefit from the arrangement. Whether overhead is reduced or there is a fundamental change to the sponsored organization, the end result is that a nonprofit is able to better help those it serves.

THE PROS AND CONS OF A SHARED GOVERNANCE MODEL

- Fiscal sponsorship is not for everyone. When deciding to work with a fiscal sponsor, it is important for a nonprofit to consider the costs and benefits that it can provide. While fiscal sponsorship can help control costs and increase organization efficiency, working with a fiscal sponsor can sometimes feel like losing autonomy.
- A nonprofit that elects to find a comprehensive fiscal sponsor often ends up becoming part of a larger organization whose leaders may be more cautious and risk averse. Depending on the nonprofit, this could be either good or bad—reduced flexibility is balanced by increased reliability.
- When nonprofits join a fiscal sponsor, their boards of directors typically transition into becoming advisory committees that control mission direction and strategic planning. This can feel like a loss of autonomy even though the groups have retained their organizational leadership. With the additional layer of oversight, leaders often express concern about being accountable to the fiscal sponsor rather than to themselves and their donors.

- However, access to stronger governance systems is in fact one of the main reasons that some nonprofits find the fiscal sponsorship model attractive. One of the most devastating problems a nonprofit can face is instability related to leadership changes and executive director turnover. The shared governance aspects of fiscal sponsorship minimize these concerns.

- Another fear that nonprofit leaders may have when considering fiscal sponsorship is the perceived loss of control. However, it is often easier to hold accountable outsourced back-office solution providers—whether a fiscal sponsor or a for-profit vendor—than it is to manage poorly performing or overworked staff. If an organization thinks its fiscal sponsor is underperforming or that independence can bring increased value to the organization, there is always the option to fire the fiscal sponsor.

- Many nonprofits fear that the services of a fiscal sponsor will be opaque. Competition in the marketplace and the need to uphold organization reputation as a best practice model keep fiscal sponsors vested in transparency and openness.

CONCLUSION

- Fiscal sponsorship, while it is underutilized in the nonprofit sector, remains an important tool for organizations that seek to make impact in their communities. Market pressures such as complex government regulations, funder restrictions, and competition for scarce resources continue to make it hard for community leaders and nonprofit executives to manage the business side of their work and, in many cases, keep their organizations alive. This trend, in combination with a greater emphasis on collaboration in the nonprofit sector, could mean that fiscal sponsorship may be of increasing value.

- The services that UAC offers to organizations with revenues of under $5 million provide a unique and valuable set of tools that are tailored to their needs and empower leaders and social entrepreneurs to solve emerging and persistent community problems.

PUT THE MONEY IN YOUR MISSION

Tivoni Devor

How Leveraging Shared Services Can Reduce the Business Costs of Running a Nonprofit

No nonprofit has a mission statement focused on managing an efficient office. You do not start a nonprofit because you are zealous about accounting, HR laws, or where you buy paper clips; nonprofits are founded to fulfill a need in the community and serve the public interest. But then there is the business of nonprofits. There is paperwork, vendor management, and millions of other little things that any small organization must deal with regardless of its mission.

Most nonprofits never rise to the scale of having a full internal administrative staff and purchased equipment. They rely on a slew of vendors for services, equipment leases, and more, but their small scales put them at a disadvantage at the negotiating table.

In the for-profit world, the business process outsourcing industry is a multibillion dollar sector that covers nearly every imaginable administrative service, and professional employer organizations are now an entire outsourcing sector that covers all HR matters. These industries provide small businesses with solutions for their common problem: How does a small organization realize an economy of scale without having the scale required?

On the nonprofit side, there are very few organizations that provide comparable services. These operational services are often provided by membership-based groups or fiscal sponsors, commonly called shared-service organizations. These organizations offer an economy of scale that they open up to other organizations, providing operational support at a price point that is more affordable than doing it internally. This allows a smaller nonprofit more flexibility in its budget to put more money in its mission.

The Benefits of Shared-Service Organizations

The above common issues are the reason that shared-service organizations have become a popular choice for new and established nonprofits to turn to for expertise and cost savings. The many costs of running any type of business, be it an LLC or a 501(c)(3), are quite similar. While they may have different funding sources, products, or services to provide, they all have to manage money, equipment, and staff.

This is where shared-service organizations can be a huge benefit for nonprofits looking to realize cost savings without compromising their programming levels; in fact, through the savings shared-service organizations generate, agencies are often able to increase their programming and help more people. Organizations such as the UAC (see previous section) in Philadelphia and other founding members of the National Network of Fiscal Sponsors (NNFS) focus on providing shared services. While any nonprofit can share services with another, members of the NNFS—Community Partners, Colorado Nonprofit Development Center, Earth Island Institute, Public Health Foundation Enterprises (PHFE) Management Solutions, Community Initiatives, Third Sector New England, and Tides—focus specifically on providing shared services at the highest standards.

For example, UAC's HR and fiscal services departments have a combined staff of 18, with specialists in nonprofit accounting, HR, benefits management, grant reporting, government contracts, payroll, and cash management. Organizations that use UAC's shared services have an assigned accountant, cloud-based online budget and accounting software, a controller, and a full C-suite to consult with, as well as other capacity-building services—systems and networks that individual organizations would find much costlier. UAC has reached its economy of scale over the last 40 years. With a collective budget of more than $25 million and more than 55 organizations and 350 employees, UAC is able, as a single entity, to negotiate with all of its vendors at a scale and create savings that the 55 individual organizations would be hard-pressed to be able to do independently. As more organizations partner with a shared-service organization, each organization's economy of scale grows, and its clients can shift even more dollars to programming.

There are many ways that an organization can find administrative savings without joining a member-based or shared-service organization. Sometimes, you just see who your neighbors are to find natural partners.

Leveraging Organic Colocation

There are many reasons that nonprofits tend to cluster. Often, it stems from multiple needs in a targeted location, but sometimes its comes down to the rent. There are several buildings in Center City Philadelphia that tend to attract nonprofit organizations for a number of reasons. One of these buildings is 1315 Walnut Street; a quick search on www.Guidestar.com pulled more than 26 nonprofits including:

The Juvenile Law Center
The Women's Business Development Center
The Energy Co-op
Girls, Inc.
Children's Aid Society
Bread and Roses Community Fund
Ten Thousand Friends of PA
Greater Philadelphia Federation
Tenant Action Group
Cultureworks
Fair Foods Philly

While these tenants vary widely in mission, scale, and size, they have more in common than a set of elevators. They all have the common need for basic business services, equipment, and administrative staff. Collectively, these 26 organizations represent several million dollars a year in administrative costs; this includes the basics such as utilities, Internet, office supplies, printers/copiers, health care, an office manager, a bookkeeper, and an accountant.

It raises some questions: Could several organizations on the same floor share a single printer/copier, office supply vendor, or office manager? How many hidden efficiencies in this building alone could create an economy of scale such that these organizations would realize savings that allowed them to increase their programming output efficiency?

Look at your organization's location. Are there other organizations located nearby with which you could colocate and potentially share services? Is your target population participating with other nonprofit organizations? Could you co-serve them?

SHOULD YOU PARTNER WITH A SHARED-SERVICE ORGANIZATION?

The principal reason to join a shared-service organization is economic. Each organization has a slightly different set of services, expertise, and fees. Shared-services fees from fiscal sponsorship organizations can range from 3% to 15% of an organization's total annual revenue depending on the services rendered. HR services are usually per employee, per month, or by percentage of total payroll. So it is important to look at your budget and compare costs to see if your organization will find an economic advantage in contracting with a shared service organization.

It is important to look at the following:

Bookkeeping and accounting costs
HR costs
Audit costs
Directors, officers, and liability insurance costs
Health insurance costs
403b and other benefit costs
Consulting costs
Executive director time spent managing the above instead of focusing on the mission

Add up these administrative costs and then calculate them as a percentage of your total budget. If that number is more than 10% of your annual budget, it is worth exploring a relationship with a shared-service organization (see Table 7.1).

As you calculate your administrative costs and your board and executive director's administrative burdens, you should also compare experience and decision-making expertise. Who would you be sharing services with? Shared services mean shared responsibilities and legally binding agreements, so when evaluating a shared-service opportunity, you should do your due diligence.

TABLE 7.1 Potential Fiscal Sponsorship Savings

Professional Service	Estimated Hourly Rate $	Illustrative # Hours per Month	Annual Cost $	As a % of a $250,000 Budget
Organizational Development	175	2.5	5,250	2.1
Economic Analysis	152	2.5	4,560	1.8
Human Resources	114	10	13,680	5.5
Financial Reporting	100	10	12,000	4.8
Tax Accountant	98	2.5	2,940	1.2
Internal Audit	97	2.5	2,910	1.2
Finance & Insurance Management	94	2.5	2,820	1.1
Management Analysis	92	2.5	2,760	1.1
Fundraising Coordinator	65	10	7,800	3.1
Total				21.9

Source: Adapted from Russell (2013).

Note: These estimated hourly rates are derived from annual salary averages for industry professionals in the Philadelphia region in each of the selected categories. An overhead rate of 2.5 and 2.0 billable hours per year are assumed.

The Scale of the Greater Philadelphia Nonprofit Sector

The five-county Philadelphia region reported more than $43 billion in revenue from a total of 17,635 nonprofits (Table 7.2). It is commonly estimated that total real nonprofit overhead is 30%, which means that in greater Philadelphia, about $13 billion goes to overhead and back-office operations: There has to be room for savings here. If every nonprofit used shared services and saved 10% in administrative costs, we could redirect $1.3 billion from overhead to programming each year (http://nccsdataweb.urban.org). Imagine that impact.

Because of many factors in the nonprofit marketplace, organizations find themselves competing more than cooperating. This dynamic

TABLE 7.2   Total Nonprofit Revenues

County	Number of Organizations Filing Form 990	Total Revenue $ Reported on Form 990
Bucks County	1,798	1,963,276,539
Chester County	2,048	2,003,247,603
Delaware County	2,046	6,337,960,046
Montgomery County	3,694	7,250,102,453
Philadelphia County	8,049	25,672,408,945
Total	17,635	43,226,995,586

Source: National Center for Charitable Statistics, Urban Institute (2012); http://nccs.urban.org/database/overview.cfm

makes shared services and colocating seem counterintuitive on the surface, but go back to your mission: Why does your nonprofit exist and how can it best be of service? Finding cost savings has the same impact as getting a cash donation. Can your organization leverage shared services, economies of scale, renegotiation, and partnership to shift 1%?

The 1% Challenge

There is no organization on the planet that cannot become 1% more efficient, and there should not be one that does not try to reduce its costs. If each one of the 17,635 area organizations became 1% more efficient, nearly $130 million would be redirected into programming, which would affect countless families and individuals in need. That works out to about $7,000 per organization, no small sum for many. As a leader in Philadelphia's nonprofit community, you should make one of your operational goals for this year to try to find these hidden efficiencies because, as we all know in Philly, a penny saved is a penny earned.

REFERENCES

Colvin, G. L. (2006a). *Fiscal sponsorship: 6 ways to do it right*. San Francisco, CA: Study Center Press.

Colvin, G. L. (2006b). *Fiscal sponsorship*. Presentation at Western Conference on Tax Exempt Organizations, Los Angeles, CA, November 17, 2006. Retrieved from www.fiscalsponsorship.com/images/WCTEO_Gregory-Colvin.pdf

Green, R., Kvaternik, J., Alarcon, I., & LaFrance Associates, LLC. (2006). *Fiscal sponsorship field scan: Understanding current needs and practices (whitepaper)*. San Francisco, CA: Tides Center. Retrieved from www.tides.org/fileadmin/user/pdf/WP_FiscalSponsorFieldScan.pdf

Leach, Mark, & Management Assistance Group, Inc. (2009). *Outsourcing back-office services in small nonprofits: Pitfalls and possibilities*. Washington, DC: Management Assistance Group, Inc. Retrieved from http://meyer-foundation.org/sites/all//files/Outsourcing-FullReport.pdf

National Center for Charitable Statistics, Urban Institute. (2012). Overview of NCCS Data Files. Retrieved from http://nccs.urban.org/database/overview.cfm

Russell, J. (2013). *Do what you do best: Outsourcing as capacity building in the nonprofit sector*. Boise, ID: Elevate Books.

Woodward, B. (2013, August 4). *How much does it cost to file for 501(c)(3) tax exemption*. Retrieved from http://nonprofitelite.com/how-much-will-it-cost-to-get-501c3-tax-exempt-2

8

Merger Myths

Thomas A. McLaughlin

EDITORS' OVERVIEW

Chapter 9 presents some examples of successful mergers in the non-profit sector, but first, in this chapter Thomas McLaughlin again offers his partnership expertise, this time to dispel some of the myths that surround nonprofit mergers.

INTRODUCTION

As the interest in nonprofit mergers grows, so do the myths surrounding them. In the nonprofit sector, mergers carry the stigma of for-profit experiences. Considering some of the legendary train wrecks that for-profit mergers have turned out to be, this is understandable; on that basis alone, many people reject them. Yet, when myths dominate thinking in place of clear-eyed analysis, decision making can get skewed. This is a good time to examine some of the more persistent ideas about mergers in the nonprofit sector.

Administrative Cost Savings

The most persistent myth about nonprofit mergers is that they will save administrative costs; maybe, but maybe not. Many well-meaning outsiders looking in on the nonprofit sector conclude that there are "too many nonprofits" and that there should be a multitude of mergers in order to save money. Mostly this myth taps into everyone's shared distaste for spending more money on administrative costs than is absolutely necessary. There is no constituency for wasteful overhead spending, so it is a risk-free proposition.

But let us look at the economic realities of nonprofits and their mergers. The vast majority of nonprofit public charities have revenues barely into six figures, and the majority rarely clear even $2 million a year. Many pressures keep administrative spending low already, so trimming even a small slice of that amount is a nearly heroic accomplishment. Those entertaining a merger with the primary idea of achieving major administrative savings will almost certainly be disappointed.

More important, any merger with the chief goal of achieving, for example, $20,000 in administrative savings is quickly going to seem like cruel and unusual punishment to those trying to make it happen. At some point, they will likely stop, look around, and ask each other "Are we doing all this just to save $20,000?" Better to have a lofty strategic goal and be realistic about administrative savings.

It is more likely that any savings will show up as more bang for the same buck. Only when one of the entities is much larger than the other, and has far more established and efficient administrative systems, will there likely be any significant administrative savings.

Fears of Massive Job Cuts

The second most pervasive myth about nonprofit mergers is that they lead to massive job losses. This fear is largely a carryover from mergers in the for-profit sector and the simplistic media coverage they usually get. Investors generally approve of mergers but they dislike the resulting dip in stock prices that they tend to bring. Chief executive officers (CEOs) need to produce a quick offset to the additional cost of the merger, and the fastest way to do that is to lay off staff. The real heart of a merger is pretty unglamorous stuff, but the local television news reporter gets a ready-made, instantly understandable story, and that becomes the lead. Interestingly, it may be the announcement itself that they are counting on to achieve the effect. One study tracked layoff announcements from the *Wall Street Journal* and calculated that if all of the announced job cuts had actually happened, the unemployment rate would have been 50%.

In the nonprofit sector, there is nothing comparable with investor pressure, so there is no inherent pressure to cut jobs. There may be incidental job losses, but any major level of job loss that occurs during a nonprofit merger was probably going to happen anyway. In fact, a merger may actually reduce some of those losses if it promotes more efficient service delivery models.

Loss of Identity

Of all the merger myths in this sector, this is one of the least understood. For practical purposes, "identity" means "brand," and managing brands is one thing that the nonprofit sector is just beginning to master. In the days when the prevailing nonprofit model was one corporation, one site, one brand, this may have been a legitimate fear. But many nonprofits are learning that it is possible and sometimes even desirable to have multiple brands under the same roof. It is important to understand that the decision to merge corporate structures is not the same thing as the decision to merge brands.

LET US FIGURE OUT THE STRUCTURE FIRST

Once the initial exploratory discussions are over, many board members and some CEOs want to jump right into a discussion about a desirable corporate structure. Big mistake; form should follow function—decide what you want the merger to accomplish and be clear about your shared assessments and desires, and only then is it worth having a discussion about the structure.

Shhhh. Do Not Tell Anyone

For-profit mergers are done in secrecy out of necessity. Large amounts of money are often made or lost on swings in stock prices, and there are laws and regulations governing what merger planners are allowed to say. Premature disclosures can sink a deal, and unauthorized outsiders (and insiders) are always willing to try to cash in on a tip.

Nonprofit mergers may well have to start out in secrecy for vaguely similar reasons. No nonprofit wants potentially damaging rumors to scare off donors or unnecessarily alarm government funders. And the wrong kind of disclosure can create unnecessary staff anxiety.

But if the best nonprofit mergers are decided from the top down, they must be implemented from the bottom up. Owning the company in a for-profit context confers "Now hear this" authority, but in the nonprofit sector, authority is diffuse, and employee buy-in and goodwill are essential for implementation.

Nonprofits can often manage the message effectively to external stakeholders such as donors and even the media. Without the lost jobs hype, nonprofit mergers take on less urgency for most media outlets. Even today, when the mainstream media picks up on stories about nonprofit mergers, the treatment tends to paint nonprofits as a monolithic industry, with specific mergers used as illustrations of broad trends rather than as the story itself.

Only Failing Organizations Merge

Ironically, this tends to be a self-fulfilling myth. If they do not clearly understand the implications of their financial conditions, many struggling nonprofits tend to hold on longer than they should. By the time they are finally ready to consider the idea, it may be too late to salvage the programs.

The result is that the first wave of mergers in a given area does tend to involve stronger organizations taking over weaker ones, so that becomes the prevailing imagery. But combining a problem-plagued organization with another, healthier organization just produces a larger organization with a lot more problems to solve. The most constructive use of mergers is not to rescue organizations in trouble—which might be done in other ways—but to strengthen community capacity by building nonprofit organizational strength.

The Increase in Mergers Is a Product of the Economic Downturn

Although it is logical to associate the increase in merger activity with the economic downturn, the fact is that many nonprofit resources are currently locked into outdated corporate structures and aging program models. While the downturn is making mergers seem like a logical choice, it is only a catalyzing agent for trends that were already under way.

In the end, mergers are simply another leadership tool. Reflexive loyalty to unneeded corporate structures or to program models in need of innovation is not a virtue. It is time to lighten the baggage of mythology.

9

Merger Case Studies

*Tine Hansen-Turton, Richard J. Cohen,
Nicholas D. Torres, Kathy Wellbank,
Joan C. Mazzotti, James Moss, Allison F. Book,
Ann O'Brien, and Carl M. Coyle*

EDITORS' OVERVIEW

For nonprofit agencies, there are generally two ways of growing: organically, which takes longer and is more detailed, or through strategic partnerships with other nonprofits. This chapter focuses on a wide range of strategic partnerships.

DEPLOYING STRATEGY TO CREATE
PURPOSEFUL PARTNERSHIPS

Tine Hansen-Turton, Richard J. Cohen, and Nicholas D. Torres

PARTNERSHIPS: FROM COLLABORATIONS TO MERGERS

Few nonprofits in the sector, other than hospitals and insurers, enter into strategic partnerships, and far fewer merge or affiliate with other nonprofits. This is in direct opposition to the private sector, in which part of business growth and development and company business plans include plans for mergers and acquisitions (M&A). Annual surveys from the Nonprofit Finance Fund have consistently shown that only a small percentage (2%–3%) of nonprofit leaders and boards, regardless of their financial positions, consider merging and affiliating with other nonprofit organizations. For every one successful nonprofit affiliation or merger, there are hundreds that did not happen but should have. Why is this? And more important, what will it take for nonprofits in the human service sector to begin to work together more strategically to consolidate operations and focus on their missions?

THE PUBLIC HEALTH MANAGEMENT CORPORATION STORY

In the wake of the Patient Protection and Affordable Care Act (ACA), the future of the health and human service sector will change dramatically. Health and human service agencies will be financially incentivized to work together. Just as managed care has taken over how health care providers are being reimbursed, the recent trend of creating managed care systems within the human service sector to take on the risk of managing foster care through the Improving Outcomes for Children initiative in Philadelphia, Pennsylvania, Florida, and Nebraska, among other places, is just the beginning of what the future will look like for traditional child and family human services.

The Public Health Management Corporation (PHMC), however, is one of the rare nonprofit health and human service organizations that has been engaged in mergers and affiliations in the past 20 years.

In this section, PHMC describes its affiliation models with a number of organizations, as well as its tips and lessons learned as a pioneer in the nonprofit health and human service affiliation and merger marketplace. Additional case studies follow, including more detailed discussions of some of the programs being presented here.

Since 1989, PHMC has strategically used its organizational infrastructure and size to partner with mission-aligned nonprofit colleagues through its affiliation model. The focus with these affiliations has mainly been on driving down costs, wrapping services around existing clients, and enabling the affiliate organizations to better focus their operational costs to better compete. PHMC has typically completed one affiliation per year. However, given the need and interest, in the past few years, it has conducted several mergers and affiliations annually.

PHMC is a Pennsylvania-based 501(c)(3) nonprofit whose mission and business model are to bring together like-minded nonprofit organizations under one parent company to collaborate with and benefit from economies of scale, information sharing, and the pooling of expertise. As a public health institute and a large nonprofit health and human service agency, PHMC creates and sustains healthier communities using best practices to improve community health through direct service, partnership, innovation, policy, research, technical assistance, and a prepared workforce.

PHMC has served greater Philadelphia since 1972 and has become one of the largest and most comprehensive health and human service organizations in the nation. It currently runs more than 250 programs that provide direct resources and care to thousands of individuals and communities across the Philadelphia metro area through its more than 350 direct services programs and 13 affiliate partner organizations, which provide behavioral health services, criminal justice services, recovery housing, emergency assistance, family services, and HIV and obesity prevention. PHMC also runs health care clinics and provides direct services to marginalized and at-risk populations such as people with HIV/AIDS, welfare recipients, children with intellectual disabilities, and the homeless. In addition, through its work in emergency preparedness across the region and its various partnerships with governments, foundations, businesses, and community-based organizations, PHMC impacts every household in the Philadelphia region. In 2013, PHMC served over 250,000 clients, and the combined annual impact of PHMC and its affiliates on the Philadelphia community's economic vitality is estimated to be in the range of $1 billion. Of every dollar received, on average 92¢—a total of $161 million—goes toward program services.

THE PHMC AFFILIATION MODEL: STRATEGIC, PURPOSEFUL PARTNERSHIP

Affiliations are strategically different from mergers. In a traditional merger, one of the organizations typically ceases to exist. Some or all staff and board leadership are absorbed into one of the organizations or into the newly merged corporate entity. Affiliations are different: In this model, staff and board leadership for the most part remain intact following some back-office consolidation. In the nonprofit sector, an affiliation is akin to the relationship between a subsidiary corporation and its parent in which the parent corporation has some level of control. In general, however, the corporations involved in affiliations operate independently but rely on economies of scale, such as through shared common back-office services (e.g., finance, human resources, information technology, and communications support).

PHMC strongly believes in the missions of its partner organizations and wants them to keep their identities and leadership as they affiliate; its management style is to stay in the background and support its affiliate organizations. The PHMC affiliation model works as follows:

- The partner agency retains its own 501(c)(3) status and federal tax identification number, files its own Internal Revenue Service (IRS) Form 990, and completes its own individual agency audit.
- The partner agency has its own board of directors and keeps its own assets and liabilities. There is a firewall between PHMC and the affiliate organization. (Chapter 10 provides a sample asset purchase and transfer agreement that includes the provision that both parties maintain their own liabilities.)
- PHMC and the partner agency sign an affiliation agreement (a sample affiliation agreement is available in Chapter 10; the chapter also offers a sample memorandum of agreement, which would be the initial document establishing between the two parties that they intend to seek an affiliation, along with a sample letter to present to the attorney general requesting approval of the partnership once agreements have been reached on both sides). The partner agency amends its articles of incorporation and bylaws to reflect the affiliation agreement and its new legal structure as a membership corporation, with PHMC as the sole member of the corporation. Built into the affiliation agreement is the ability for the two organizations to part ways should the partnership not flourish.
- Existing partner agency staff are retained, but human resources (HR) policies and benefits are changed to better mirror those of PHMC.

- Existing board members remain on the partner agency's board, but PHMC also appoints two members. PHMC also has a seat for affiliate board representation on its own board.
- Following a due diligence process that analyzes the partner organization's need for back-office support, the partner agency enters into an annual management contract (a sample management agreement is available in Chapter 10) with PHMC for PHMC's provision of information systems, fiscal services, human resources, communications and marketing, program and strategy development, quality assurance, and related infrastructure services with an arm's length negotiated service contract.

This innovative affiliation model has allowed PHMC to create a nonprofit health system with far-reaching scope, and Chapter 10 offers an affiliation feasibility assessment for use in determining whether a potential partner is a good fit for an affiliation.

Why Should Nonprofit Organizations Affiliate?

With the recent implementation of the ACA, the health and human service landscape will change as we know it in the next decade. There are tremendous challenges and opportunities on the horizon, and one could speculate that there will be less of a need for traditional human services once all aspects of health care reform have been implemented. However, each side of the sector needs the other. As an example, for a newly insured adult in an underserved community to be healthy, access to good physical health through the ACA will not be enough. The other traditional human service supports—for example, case workers who assist and empower individuals, groups, families, and communities to prevent, alleviate, or better cope with crisis, change, and stress to enable them to function more effectively in all areas of life and living—will be essential to ensuring good health. Health care practice is rather narrow, whereas the human service sector uses a broader model to assess and deliver services. This model views people, services, and the social environment as integrated entities, a perspective that helps individuals, families, and communities address and overcome the challenges and barriers that arise from the wide range of social problems and adverse societal conditions. The sooner health and human service agencies realize they need each other, the more successful both will be in the future.

For any affiliation to be successful, the process starts with the support of both the senior leadership and the board members of both organizations. This is key to the success of these strategic partnerships. PHMC has built its model around attracting agencies that are mission aligned and whose services can be wrapped around existing consumers within the PHMC family. Furthermore, PHMC believes strongly that there is strength in numbers and that through affiliation, both organizations can have broader community impact. However, there are some key strategic indicators that should be in play before considering an affiliation. Both agencies should have the same goals in mind and should ask themselves the following key questions: Would this affiliation

- strengthen existing compatible missions?
- increase opportunities to preserve critical community assets and extend the programs offered by both organizations?
- enhance financial stability and create economies of scale?
- strengthen program and operations infrastructure capacity?
- grow new relationships that will support each organization's mission?
- provide new opportunities for staff career advancement and benefits, as well as access to academic programs and training to retain talent?

In PHMC's case, the affiliate organization's leadership is typically looking for specific opportunities and is looking to grow and scale. Primarily, they want

- Access to a network of new partners, clients, and funders
- Access to new sources of philanthropic and public funding
- The ability to bid on and secure larger private and public contracts by having the backing of a larger parent organization
- Administrative and infrastructure support as needed, including but not limited to human resources, information technology, accounting, and marketing

- The ability to accelerate the growth of existing programs, services and markets, and to enter new markets
- Access to a line of credit

THE AFFILIATION PROCESS—HOW IT WORKS

PHMC's affiliation process typically takes up to 6 months of mutual organizational due diligence. In the first 2 months, PHMC's affiliation team meets with the prospective affiliate partner's board and leadership to determine the interest in exploring an affiliation. Prior to the formal process, PHMC would have already conducted preliminary analysis of the nonprofit's financial health. One of the challenges in the nonprofit sector is that often when an organization's leadership begins to think about strategic partnerships, the organization has begun to lose money. But by the time that has happened, it is almost always too late to initiate the process.

Once there is overall leadership support, both parties sign a nondisclosure agreement (see Chapter 10 for a sample). Over a 60-day period, both agencies complete a mutual programmatic and fiscal due diligence analysis. As a management company, PHMC specifically focuses its efforts on assessing back-office support needs and developing management contracts, based on the organization's needs in the areas of human resources, information systems, and finance support. Because its management services are needs-based, PHMC is generally more competitive compared with agencies that charge a flat back-office overhead rate. Over the 60- to 120-day due diligence period, program staff explore program development opportunities, including funders and contracts. PHMC also analyzes the potential impact of the affiliation on other affiliates and partners. In this period, the affiliation agreement is negotiated, quality management issues are identified, and marketing and communication strategies are developed. Finally, in the 120- to 180-day period, both boards finalize the approval of the affiliation agreement and the change of bylaws and complete and sign the management contract. Staff of the affiliate partner organization are introduced to the transition plan. All administrative issues for on-board and ongoing maintenance are finalized, such as consolidating human resource policies and financial management, including accounts payable, billing, and purchasing arrangements, and integrating information systems.

The affiliation process can end at any given point during the 6-month period. The process typically ends based on board and leadership discomfort with parent-control issues and when it is obvious that the missions are not aligned and the parties have fewer prospects than initially believed. Nevertheless, while the due diligence process is key to successful affiliations, the leadership of both organizations take a leap of faith that the partnership will bear fruit for both.

Affiliation Impact and Why Relationships Matter

To date, all PHMC affiliate organizations have increased their budgets and community impact up to tenfold or more within a short period: The wholes have clearly been greater than the sums of their parts.

Contrary to M&A in the private sector, nonprofit sector mergers and affiliations are a relationship business. The common theme behind the success of all of the affiliations is relationships, built on trust and over time. These include relationships between PHMC's and the affiliate organization's leaderships as well as in the funding community, including the City of Philadelphia, which has a vested interest in ensuring that the organizations it supports are strong fiscally and in management.

PHMC is no different. The following summaries tell background stories of relationships among leadership and staff that have been built over time and on a foundation of trust.

Interim House

Interim House (IH) was PHMC's first venture into the affiliation model; Richard J. Cohen had a strong relationship with the organization and its leadership. IH services were known to be considered exceptional by the women served in the residential treatment facility in Mt. Airy. However, the organization and program were in financial distress. Funding agencies such as Philadelphia's offices of substance abuse and drugs and alcohol were very supportive of PHMC's helping the program, which started with PHMC entering into a management contract to turn the agency around. PHMC provided management services with support from city government agencies, and the board ultimately turned into an affiliation in 1989, eventually creating a program for women and their children at IH West in West Philadelphia. However, it was the relationships that PHMC's leadership had with the organization and the funding community, including the city, that enabled the affiliation to happen.

The Bridge

In the early 1990s, The Bridge, a residential program for adolescents, was in such serious financial trouble that it was at risk of going out of business. The program was strong and well-liked by funders such as the City of Philadelphia, but it was losing significant amounts of money. PHMC was retained with support from the city's drug and alcohol office to do a management intervention. When PHMC intervened in 1993, the program was losing over $500,000/year. PHMC and its lawyers did something unheard of in the nonprofit sector at that time yet common in the private sector: It put Bridge through bankruptcy in order to resolve all of its debt issues. PHMC negotiated with all of Bridge's creditors and came to a common agreement on payback terms for funding earned, and within a 6-month period, the debt was resolved. The Bridge became an affiliate of PHMC in 1994 and became a PHMC subsidiary organization. Since then, the agency has been well-managed within a fee-for-service environment and with strong leadership and is set to grow in the coming years.

Health Promotion Council

The former executive director of Health Promotion Council (HPC) had been a long-time colleague and friend of PHMC's president and other senior management. However, the affiliation idea was initiated by a Philadelphia-region consultant, who introduced HPC's leadership to thinking about possibly affiliating with a larger mission-aligned organization that could help it grow and scale. HPC affiliated in 1999 and has seen tremendous growth and expansion in services through the affiliation, including its ability to successfully bid on state funding, which it would not have been able to secure without a strong infrastructure such as PHMC's. Most recently, another PHMC affiliate, Resources for Children's Health, consolidated its programs with HPC and now operates as an HPC program.

National Nursing Centers Consortium

PHMC manages a network of nurse-managed federally qualified health centers and was a founding member of what eventually became the National Nursing Centers Consortium (NNCC) in 1996—there was complete mission alignment from the beginning. In 2001, what had been the board of the Regional Nursing Centers Consortium, and the chief executive officer (CEO) who ran it, decided to go national and focus on the key policy and program issues of the nurse-managed health center movement. The focus on policy and programs led the group to easily decide that affiliating with an organization with strong infrastructure and back-office support would be key to its success, as well as to its need to focus on the national and state policies that affected nurse practitioners and nurse-managed health clinics. As with most affiliations, the rubber hits the road when organizations begin to discuss control and ownership. In an affiliate model, the parent organization is the legal owner. However, NNCC and PHMC leadership came to an agreement that there should be an exit clause in the affiliation agreement in case the partnership should not work out. NNCC affiliated in 2002 and has seen tremendous organizational growth while helping to transform how primary care is delivered in the United States, and the organization has raised more than $300 million nationally on behalf of its members. The affiliation model was key to NNCC's success in focusing on its true mission.

The Joseph J. Peters Institute

PHMC's president and CEO and its former board chair were both on the Joseph J. Peters Institute (JJPI) board. After a 5-year period of discussing the possibility of affiliating, both the Office of Mental Health and the Office of Community Behavioral Health approved of the affiliation, which took place in 2004.

Metropolitan Career Center

Metropolitan Career Center (MCC), one of the region's most respected workforce and associate's degree programs, affiliated with PHMC in 2011. The affiliation came about through a relationship between the former executive director and PHMC's president and CEO. MCC's executive director was very well aware that the organization would need to close its doors without the support of an organization like PHMC. At this time, PHMC is in the process of turning the organization around, adding degrees such as allied health as well as growing the workforce programs.

Turning Points for Children

Turning Points for Children's (TPFC) CEO and both PHMC's president and CEO and its chief strategy officer (CSO), had known each other for years. With the change in human services toward community-based interventions, it became clear to TPFC's CEO that he would need to partner with more diverse nonprofits. Specifically, he was looking for a leadership team that was entrepreneurial and had an eye toward the opportunities (and challenges) of the future. TPFC joined PHMC on February 1, 2013, with the intent to operationalize the natural synergies between its prevention and child welfare services and PHMC's medical and behavioral health services. This affiliation enabled TPFC to offer more comprehensive and coordinated child and family services.

Lessons Learned From the PHMC Affiliation Model

As with all partnerships, relationships built on trust are critical to success. Some of these relationships take years to build, so patience is key. The affiliation process can be taxing on the staffs of both organizations, so it is important that the leadership be serious. In PHMC's case, its affiliation focus tends to be on organizations that have annual budgets of $3 million or more. The process generally starts with the leadership of both organizations connecting and coming to trust that a strategic alliance is the right way to go based on substantial and thorough due diligence. Mission alignment is critical, and so is the leadership of the partner organization. As critical as mission is, so is the belief that the partnership will increase opportunities to preserve critical community assets and extend the programs offered by both organizations. The enhanced financial stability and newly created economies of scale, particularly in administration and infrastructure, are equally critical. Finally, career advancement opportunities are also relevant to retaining nonprofit organizational talent.

Outside agencies such as local governments and foundations can play important roles in the affiliation process, from encouraging nonprofits to affiliate or merge to investing critical juncture funding to support the due diligence and implementation phases of the affiliation. One misconception is that affiliations are operationally cheaper, but that is not necessarily true (although PHMC can demonstrate that to date, all of its affiliate organizations have been able to drive down overhead costs over time through creating economies of scale). PHMC has been appreciative over the years of the past support of local government agencies in encouraging affiliations, as well as that of funders such as The Philadelphia Foundation, United Way, and the Independence Foundation that provided critical juncture funding. More of this kind of leadership is needed to encourage more of these strategic partnerships.

Affiliate Program Profiles in Order of Year of Affiliation

Interim House (1989)

IH is a corporation licensed by the Commonwealth of Pennsylvania's Bureau of Drug and Alcohol Programs. The center provides a continuum of comprehensive services to women addicted to drugs and alcohol that comprises three levels of care: residential treatment, intensive outpatient treatment, and outpatient counseling. Incorporated in 1971, IH was the first such specialized program in the Commonwealth of Pennsylvania and one of the first in the nation, and it has served as a model for the innovative treatment of substance-abusing women. IH utilizes a holistic, trauma-sensitive approach to treating drug and alcohol addiction that focuses on the physical, mental, emotional, and spiritual issues surrounding addiction. It offers a wide range of therapeutic and support services, with an emphasis on preventing relapse, establishing stability and responsibility, improving life and parenting skills, and developing and strengthening support systems and links to support services.

The Bridge (1994)

Since 1971, The Bridge has helped over 10,000 people challenged by addictions. The primary goal of The Bridge is to provide quality, accessible treatment while preparing clients to reenter their communities as drug- and alcohol-free members of society. The Bridge understands that individuals who have become dependent on alcohol and/or other drugs frequently experience many other problems. Their treatment philosophy stresses a holistic approach; interventions focus on treating the addiction, its underlying causes, and its related dysfunctions.

The Bridge offers a range of services designed to meet the needs of persons of all ages with addiction-related issues. The program serves adolescents from neighborhoods throughout Philadelphia, the suburban counties, and the state of Delaware. The Bridge offers long- and short-term residential programs for up to 38 adolescents and outpatient counseling for children, adolescents, and adults. Individualized treatment plans are created to meet clients' needs, and clients have access to comprehensive addiction, mental health, education, and life skills services.

HPC and Resources for Children's Health (1999)

HPC is a nonprofit corporation that was organized in 1981. Its mission is to promote health and prevent and manage chronic diseases, especially among vulnerable populations, through community-based outreach, education, and advocacy. Its unique programs advocating positive health behaviors, together with its innovative work with minority groups, have advanced the field of health promotion in southeastern Pennsylvania and across the nation. As part of its mission to promote health and provide outreach and education, HPC conducts family support and healthy parenting education programs, including its Health Intervention Program and Focus on Families, formerly available through Resources for Children's Health. HPC has a diverse, multicultural, multilingual staff and fulfills its mission through programs in four major areas: chronic disease risk reduction; chronic disease prevention and management; community and capacity building; and professional education and consulting.

NNCC (2002)

NNCC, the leading advocate for nurse-managed health care, is a nonprofit corporation whose mission is to strengthen the capacity, growth, and development of nurse-managed health centers, provide quality care to vulnerable populations, and eliminate health disparities in underserved communities. NNCC advocates for accessible health care provided by nurses as the primary care providers (PCPs). Its nurse-run member health centers provide community-based care that is sensitive to patient needs and concerns. NNCC works to improve policies for nurse practitioners as PCPs and also helps member health centers meet the costs of providing care to the uninsured and underinsured by taking the lead in developing and running programs in partnership with its member centers that help people lead healthier and safer lives. These programs help avert future health problems and keep health care costs from rising.

JJPI (2004)

JJPI is a nonprofit mental health agency that provides outpatient sexual abuse assessment and treatment services. JJPI's mission is to reduce the causes and overall impact and outcomes of sexually abusive behaviors through research, training, prevention, and treatment. The Institute evaluates and treats survivors of sexual abuse as well as offenders. In addition, JJPI provides training to organizations throughout the region and has a national reputation for its work in sexual abuse assessment, treatment, prevention, and education. Its research arm has received numerous grants from foundations such as the National Institutes of Health and the National Institute of Justice.

MCC (2011)

MCC was launched in 1974 as a nonprofit workforce development organization established by the clergy and members of the First United Methodist Church of Germantown to help neighborhood youth and adults gain greater access to resources that could lead to better careers and higher education. Today, MCC and its nonprofit career school, Computer Technology Institute (CTI), educate and train individuals who have limited access to resources to connect them to employers and help meet changing workforce needs. MCC and CTI encourage sustainable careers and economic independence by building a supportive learning environment in which students receive personalized attention. To further that mission, CTI, an approved and accredited training provider through the Department of Education and one of the few nonprofit secondary career schools in Pennsylvania, offers an associate's degree in specialized technology and a diploma in health information technology.

TPFC (2013)

TPFC serves approximately 2,500 families and 5,700 children per year through a range of prevention and intervention programs. The agency was initially created in 2008, when the Children's Aid Society of Pennsylvania (CASPA) merged with the Philadelphia Society for Services to Children (PSSC). CASPA and PSSC—both small organizations similar in size, mission, and programming—chose to merge in order to become one organization with a stronger infrastructure and more sustainable resources. This merger proved to be successful in that the organization operated more efficiently, was better able to attract public and private funding, and had an enhanced portfolio of outcome-based services through which to serve vulnerable children and families. (The details of the merger between PSSC and CASPA will be discussed in more detail in the "Turning Points for Children" section later in this chapter.) Before the merger, PSSC and CASPA had nearly 300 years of collective experience serving youth and families. For many decades, the services were primarily related to placement (foster care, group homes, residential treatment, and adoption). With the beginning of family support strategies in the early 1970s, the agencies began to provide in-home and community-based services. TPFC uses its resources to serve those struggling with the effects of chronic poverty: difficult family relationships, domestic violence, substance abuse, child abuse and neglect, teen pregnancy, poor education and high dropout rates, unemployment, substandard housing, and inadequate health care. The goal is not simply to prevent negative outcomes but to help families recognize and act on their strengths, helping them reach their greatest potential by identifying and achieving their individual and family goals. Throughout TPFC's programming, there is a long history of effectively working with children, youth, and families to enable them to develop the skills they need to set and achieve goals, overcome obstacles, locate and utilize community resources, advocate for themselves, and develop stability, healthy lifestyles, and productive futures. TPFC is accredited by the Council on Accreditation and is a member of the Alliance for Children and Families and the Pennsylvania Council for Children, Youth and Family Services.

The Villa (2013)

The Villa is a specialized residential program for youth that serves young people with a history of truancy, emotional trauma, family conflict, and difficulties in the community; it partners with The Bridge, another PHMC affiliate. Villa nurtures growth, teaches responsibility, and restores hope among its residents. Its mission is to empower children and families through strong community collaborations and to teach them to lead responsible lives and develop healthy relationships. The Villa's comprehensive program addresses the physical, cognitive, social, educational, and emotional needs of youth so they can become productive members of society. It offers services to address academic issues, strengthen family relationships, and develop age-appropriate social skills. Additionally, the programming focuses on the skill development necessary for reunification with family and introduction into the public school system. The Villa, formerly St. Mary's Villa for Children and Families, was founded in 1911 as an orphanage for boys by the sisters of the Holy Family of Nazareth. In 1936, the orphanage moved to the spacious, historic grounds of the Lindenwold Estate in Ambler, Pennsylvania. In 2001, St. Mary's Villa combined resources with Holy Family Institute in Pittsburgh and developed a reputation as a preeminent provider of services for abused and neglected children in greater Philadelphia.

The Villa serves both boys and girls in need of care and an opportunity for a fresh start. Services are also available through their day school for students from surrounding school districts who need special education services.

INNOVATIONS THROUGH PARTNERSHIPS IN RECOVERY: A CASE STUDY OF PHMC'S IH

Kathy Wellbank and Devin Reaves

SUMMARY

The City of Philadelphia faces dire straits. Both nationwide and specifically in Pennsylvania, social services and assistance programs designed to bolster those battling substance use disorders are being slashed in a city that is infested with open-air drug markets and widespread poverty. With 33% of the women of Philadelphia living below the poverty level, finding adequate resources to serve their varied needs is a difficult task. In 1989, Interim House, Inc. and PHMC came together in what was then and is still today considered an innovative way to partner through affiliating to operate the oldest women-only substance abuse treatment center in Pennsylvania and one of the first on the East Coast. More than a decade later, this partnership has helped create an innovative program that has been recognized around the city and the country as a leader and model for trauma-informed, gender-specific addiction treatment. Kathy Wellbank, the director of the program, attributed the program's success to its affiliation with PHMC. This affiliation provided with her the time to create a vision and the tools to implement, manage, and grow the program. In conversation, she attested that without the support and expertise of the PHMC team, she would be bogged down completing tedious reports and writing grants that would take her away from keeping her finger on the pulse of the program's changing needs and creating programs to meet these needs. She expressed much enthusiasm over the importance of PHMC staff's mirroring the director's philosophy and leadership traits in making the partnership so successful, and stated that she owes her ability to thrive in this leadership role to the talent and expertise of PHMC, who also demonstrate positive leadership qualities such as integrity, dedication, creativity, fairness, openness, humility, and a sense of humor. She particularly emphasized the importance of trust, collective talent and teamwork, compassion, stability, and relationships in her interactions with PHMC. Without trust and these excellent working relationships, the affiliation would not be successful. The program director emphasized that effective leaders, such as those at PHMC, are able to surround themselves with the right people, who have not only the education and skills to perform their jobs but also the emotional intelligence to work well with and adjust to the varying personalities and changing conditions they will encounter.

PHMC plays a critical role for IH in strategic planning, board development, fundraising, contract monitoring, human resources, fiscal services, billing and accounting management, information technology, and grant writing. Being part of a corporation that provides public health services to various populations has also helped create a synergy for sharing information with and learning from the expertise of others in similar management positions.

As with many of PHMC's affiliate organizations, IH has grown and flourished with the assistance of PHMC since its affiliation in 1989. IH provides first-rate clinical services to the low-income underinsured/ uninsured recovering women in Philadelphia and in other counties in Pennsylvania. Insight into the affiliation model is exemplified in the case study of IH and in the story of Virginia, an alumna of this historic program.

BACKGROUND ON SUBSTANCE ABUSE

Substance abuse is a complex problem that, like many other social problems, is complicated to navigate, and relevant interventions are hard to implement. Substance abuse is defined by the American Psychiatric Association (APA) as "a maladaptive pattern of substance use leading to clinically significant impairment or distress as manifested by one (or more) of the following [criteria], occurring within a 12-month period," including "recurrent substance use resulting in a failure to fulfill major role obligations at work, school, or home (such as repeated absences or poor work performance related to substance use), recurrent substance use in situations in which it is physically hazardous (such as driving an automobile or operating a machine when impaired by substance use), recurrent substance-related legal problems" (APA, 2000, p. 199). The APA further defines the impact on individuals as including "tolerance, withdrawal, a persistent desire or unsuccessful efforts to cut down or control substance use, a great deal of time is spent in activities necessary to obtain the substance, use the substance, or recover from its effects, important social, occupational, or recreational activities are given up or reduced because of substance use" (APA, 2000, p. 197). Treating this population is difficult, and it drains limited resources.

Public services for individuals in Philadelphia suffering from substance abuse disorders have been lacking since the crack epidemic of the 1980s. All major urban centers including New York and Chicago were underequipped and undereducated to handle this sweeping drug. As this powerful stimulant was hitting the streets of Philadelphia in the early 1980s, we met Virginia. Virginia was a 16-year-old African American teenager born in South Philadelphia. By her 16th birthday, Virginia was already a single mother and experimenting with speed pills, alcohol, and benzodiazepines (medications normally prescribed for anxiety disorders). By the time Virginia was 17 years old, she had become a sex worker at a nude modeling studio to survive and to finance her drug habit. In just a few years, the crack cocaine began to take its toll on Virginia's life, and she was forced out of the modeling studio, winding up working the streets of North Philadelphia for a fraction of her previous rate. At this point, Virginia had several arrests for prostitution and drug possession and had become estranged from her family and young child.

In this same era, IH was already over a decade old and struggling to keep its doors open. IH was founded by Clara Baxter Synigal, an

African American woman and recovering alcoholic who realized the importance of gender-specific treatment owing to her personal experience with treatment for alcoholism and the difficulty she experienced when sharing sensitive issues in mixed-gender programs. At its inception, IH was one of the first women-only substance-abuse facilities in the country. With the economic downturn of the 1980s and the introduction of crack cocaine, IH was overwhelmed. With only a single revenue stream to depend on, the City of Philadelphia, its outlook was bleak. In 1989, IH became an affiliate of PHMC (then Philadelphia Health Management Corporation) to keep its doors open. The executive director of IH, Kathy Wellbank, describes this as a turning point for the agency.

Over the next 15 years, everything changed for IH. With the assistance of PHMC, including its infrastructure and back-office support, IH was able to diversify its revenue streams, receiving grants from a variety of public and private organizations over the years. Sources included the Pew Charitable Trusts and donations from United Way of southeastern Pennsylvania. These donations and grants also expanded the clinical services offered, and IH also received funding to provide psychiatric services to its clientele. The offering of psychiatric services alongside drug and alcohol counseling is key for clients with co-occurring mental health issues. Without these services, women at IH could experience undiagnosed mental health issues that would lead to relapse and failed recovery attempts. During this same time period, through the leadership and guidance of PHMC, IH received funding from the Philadelphia Department of Human Services (DHS) for services to be provided to the children of mothers in IH programs. Each of these additions is indicative of an agency evolving with the speed of research to provide cutting-edge clinical services to its patients and a dynamic family program driven by sound resource development.

Substance abuse affects not only the identified patients but also the people around the user. Substance abuse within the family unit can also have profound effects on other members of the household, especially children. These children face biological, psychological, and environmental risk. The effects on the children of family substance abuse are not isolated to the children who live with the abuser. Even children who do not still live with the substance abuser face a number of stressors (Barnard & McKeganey, 2004). When there is intensive drug use in the home, there is always the risk of poor hygiene, lack of proper child supervision, and lapses in child health care. These are frightening facts considering that over 6 million children younger than 18 years live with at least one parent who is dependent on alcohol or drugs (SAMHSA report finds 6 million children live with addicted parents, 2003).

Meanwhile, back in the early 2000s, while PHMC and IH were enjoying growth through their strategic partnership, Virginia's story went from bad to worse. She was arrested a dozen times, served jail terms in county and state prisons, overdosed seven times, and had four failed attempts at sobriety. Her fourth attempt was possibly the most dramatic and traumatic. Virginia was still a sex worker in North Philadelphia, working with undesirable characters to set up and rob johns. An empathetic police officer who knew her chased away a would-be john/victim and convinced her to go to the hospital and get some help. While at the hospital, Virginia was shocked to find out that she was pregnant and that it was quite possible that her unborn child was also addicted to the illicit drugs she was using. Virginia began a methadone maintenance program because the symptoms of withdrawal from opiates (such as heroin) can cause miscarriage. After 18 months drug-free, Virginia experienced a crushing relapse, losing again her relationships with her family and her two children. By 2006, Virginia was back on the streets, addicted to drugs and soon back in the criminal justice system.

The very next year, in 2007, staff grant writers at PHMC helped IH obtain a grant from the Pew Fund Capacity Building Program. The Pew funding allowed IH to implement a comprehensive, evidence-based training and supervision model to help clients manage their feelings, urges, and behaviors constructively (Linehan, 1994). Integrating dialectical behavioral therapy (DBT) techniques into the agency's clinical practices helped meet the needs of the increasing number of women with serious mental health disorders. With this increased clinical capacity, IHI was able to improve its clients' clinical outcomes, increase its staff's clinical knowledge and capacity, and reduce the stresses experienced by staff in working with these high-acuity clients. The program was so successful after its first year that it has since expanded to include ancillary and clinical staff.

IH also quadrupled its resource stream, receiving funding not only from the Pew Charitable Trust and United Way but also Woman's Way, the Genauridi Family Foundation, The Barra Foundation, The Northwest Foundation, and the Patricia Kind Family Foundation. IH is now an innovative agency providing first-rate services. Also in 2007, Virginia was making another attempt at recovery; after spending another year of her life in the Philadelphia corrections system, she was paroled to the new and improved IH.

At IH, Virginia was treated by master's-level clinicians, and a psychiatrist discovered an underlying diagnosis of depression. At the time, IH was offering a step-down outpatient program through which clients who discharged from the program could return a few nights a week to continue clinical services. Virginia credits IH with teaching her the tools she needed to be successful in the world. She took advantage of every program that IH offered, including faith-based services that she said increased her engagement with and outlook on life. Virginia is a woman who had been arrested 19 times in her life, yet after only 6 months at IH, she described herself as a new woman. Now almost 6 years sober, she works as an IH peer specialist. She strives to share her experiences, strength, and hope with the women at IH hoping to be the program's next success story.

PHMC and IH, through their affiliation, were instrumental in providing the support needed to help save Virginia's life. PHMC's model to affiliate with nonprofit-aligned businesses dates back more than a decade, with IH being the first to affiliate. Unlike nonprofit mergers, in the affiliation model PHMC has adopted each organization retains its own 501(c)(3) status and federal tax ID number and files its own IRS Form 990 and audit. When a new agency affiliates with PHMC, existing agency staff are usually retained, and human relations policies are modified to match PHMC standards. Existing board members are retained, and two PHMC board members are appointed. A number of infrastructure systems are added to affiliate agencies, including consolidation into a single-pay master system, information technology, and marketing and branding.

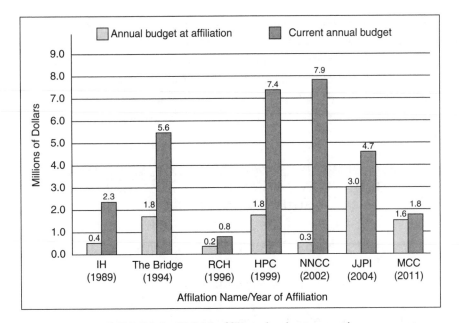

FIGURE 9.1   PHMC affiliate budget growth.
HPC, Health Promotion Council; IH, Interim House;
JJPI, Joseph J. Peters Institute; NNCC, National Nursing Centers Consortium;
MCC, Metropolitan Career Center; RCH, Resources for Children's Health.

To date, the PHMC affiliation model has proven to be fairly effective. Most of the nonprofits that have affiliated (seven to date) have seen their budgets increase five- and sixfold. PHMC operates other agencies with less than 7% overhead and has a solid management and back-office infrastructure to support these affiliate nonprofits. Figure 9.1 shows the budget growth for some of PHMC's affiliates over the years.

CONCLUSION

The PHMC affiliation model could easily be replicated anywhere. The parent company structure with several affiliates creates an ecosystem in which the sum of the parts is greater than the whole. It is possible for any large nonprofit to utilize the affiliation model to expand its community impact and to help the nonprofit organizations in its vicinity. Providing each affiliate with expertise in a variety of areas that a typical single agency would never afford, could be a boon to any agency. Experienced professionals from PHMC help affiliated agencies that wish to continue as relevant operations with program evaluation, needs assessments, strategic planning, and all key practices. Ultimately, through affiliation, both organizations can have broader community impact, and therein lies the social innovation.

AN INNOVATIVE APPROACH TO COLLABORATION: UNITED WAY OF GREATER PHILADELPHIA AND SOUTHERN NEW JERSEY

Allison F. Book and Ann O'Brien

BACKGROUND

United Way of Greater Philadelphia and Southern New Jersey (UWGPSNJ) was recently formed by merging seven regional United Ways: Atlantic, Burlington, Camden, Cape May, and Cumberland counties in New Jersey and, in Pennsylvania, Southeast Delaware County and Southeastern Pennsylvania. UWGPSNJ's mission is "to harness, leverage and strategically invest the collective power of donors, advocates and volunteers, to drive measurable results that improve the lives of people in our region." The regional United Ways recognized that by leveraging their collective strengths and developing a more cohesive message, they could develop and deliver a common donor experience and more strategically and effectively move from being grant makers to engaging local communities in making real change across the region. The ability to scale up while maintaining local presence and meeting local community needs evolved through initial exploratory conversations into a collaborative process that resulted in a decision to merge on July 1, 2012. While each United Way was individually successful at meeting its local needs, delivering on the collective brand promise was difficult. After months of thoughtful conversation and planning, the groundwork was laid, meaningful trust was established, and merging seven United Ways into one large regional organization to collectively deliver one cohesive and consistent message—while meeting local community needs and capitalizing on local relationships—became possible. Through this unique collective process, this successful merger and its expected trajectory toward sustainability make it a promising model for national replication.

Nonprofit mergers are increasing in prevalence for various reasons. Many nonprofits are merging because they are serving similar populations or providing similar services and through merging they can reduce back-office costs (La Piana, 2010). Environmental factors such as increased organizational competition or decreased foundation or donor funding encourage nonprofits to contemplate mergers (Dewey & Kaye, 2007). Because of the current economic downturn, there is increased competition for more scarce financial resources. When nonprofits with similar missions choose to merge, capacity to compete successfully for limited funding streams and donations can increase. Yet will that alone suffice to ensure the success of the surviving organization?

The merger among the seven regional United Ways is an example of a successful one. This merger demonstrates that a positive union can result from financially and programmatically viable organizations when approached from a position of strength, collaboration, and trust. The new regional United Way will continue to focus on strategies to drive lasting change in education, income, and health while working toward providing greater breadth and depth of programming in local communities over the long term.

These seven local United Ways engaged in a very thoughtful and deliberate process through strategic dialogue and conversation, considering varying factors such as local decision-making processes and key volunteer, donor, and corporate relationships. Thus, they were more prepared to prosper once the merger was completed because they understood many of the issues they would need to address to support their continued success. This deliberate process can provide insight for other organizations that are interested in learning about and potentially designing effective mergers aimed at increasing organizational efficiency, improving programs, and delivering collective and collaborative results.

INTRODUCTION

United Ways throughout the country work to ensure that all children, families, and seniors have access to quality education, a family-sustaining income, and good health (http://unitedforimpact.org/our-impact). While the means used to achieve these goals may differ slightly in each community, the goals are the same.

In Greater Philadelphia and Southern New Jersey, United Way prepares children to successfully enter kindergarten through its Success by 6® program, designed to improve the quality of early childhood education centers, provide access to these high-quality programs to low-income families, and offer parent and caregiver support and education (http://unitedforimpact.org/our-impact/education/early-childhood-education/success-by-6). United Way continues that investment in education throughout a child's academic career, focusing on early literacy to ensure that kids can read at grade level, intervening in middle and high school through innovative mentoring programs to make sure kids graduate, and providing exposure to higher education and the workplace—as well as the support to get there—so that young adults continue on to college (http://unitedforimpact.org/our-impact/education).

United Way also supports working individuals and their families. By equipping workers with job training and the financial knowledge they need to build assets and savings to provide for their family's future, they will also be empowered to contribute back to our community and economy (http://unitedforimpact.org/our-impact/income). And, of course, health is essential for thriving at home, at school, and at work. To help children, families, and seniors achieve and maintain health, United Way connects individuals and families with the resources they need to make healthy choices by investing in programs that fight barriers to health such as childhood obesity, substance abuse behaviors, and lack of access to healthy meals (http://unitedforimpact.org/our-impact/health).

United Ways throughout the Delaware Valley began meeting several years ago to discuss how to best collaborate to expand their impact. Conversations began through informal dialogue on how to come together on the national issues of education, health, and income. Through strategic conversations and the exchange of ideas, five local United Ways in New Jersey and two in Pennsylvania began to discuss the possibility of a merger in order to create a stronger, more robust presence in the region.

THE ISSUE

By 2010, most nonprofits, including United Ways in the Delaware Valley, were facing increasingly complex social problems, competing for limited resources, and learning to do more with less. Most notably, a changing and progressively more complex landscape meant: (a) regional live–work patterns across county and state lines meant donors were receiving different United Way messages from differing solicitations coming to the workplace versus home and (b) the region's needs were becoming more pressing and local United Ways needed to move from making grants to making change across the region.

United Ways have conducted much of their fundraising in the workplace. The region has shifted from having a significant donor base concentrated among corporations to a less heavily headquartered region (Adams, Bartelt, Elesh, & Goldstein, 2008). As an increasing number of nonprofit workplaces (such as hospitals and universities) have been growing and trying to raise their own funds, maintaining their support bases has become increasingly challenging. Fundraising strategies have also shifted to focus on small and mid-sized businesses, which are on the rise. In addition, the population shift away from urban areas has resulted in the upsurge of the "bedroom suburb" phenomenon, which has made it challenging for United Way to deliver a cohesive and consistent message throughout the region. These United Ways operated within the shared media market of Greater Philadelphia, with many donors commuting across multiple United Way service areas, resulting in a confusing, "noisy," and often fragmented United Way experience. In order to make sense to and potentially attract new partners and engage new volunteers, these United Ways needed a different business model to design and deliver a clear, consistent, collective message and brand promise while mitigating the declining workplace-centered fundraising trends.

Historically, United Way was an umbrella of agencies, raising dollars and allocating them to community pots for local organizations to apply. Yet over the last several years, regional United Ways have changed, moving toward making significant, long-lasting changes locally as well as impacting community conditions, particularly in education, income, and health. Although all regional United Ways had established the need to move toward a more outcomes-based model, they were all in different places in shifting from being grant makers to change makers. As United Way moved toward driving greater regional change, many realized that they were unable to do that alone working county by county.

Lastly, with the region expecting one of the worst financial crises since the Great Depression, the need for services throughout the area was pressing. With high unemployment rates, increasing poverty rates, and greater demand for services from local agencies, the demand in turn for United Way funding was even greater.

THE SOLUTION: REGIONALIZATION

The Initial Conversation

United Ways in and around Philadelphia have partnered through a group called United Ways of Delaware Valley for over a quarter century. These United Ways knew that their infrastructures were thinly resourced but that they had a lot in common, particularly in approach, vision alignment, and commitment to bringing about positive change in local communities. As conversations progressed, leaders came to believe there might be a way to restructure their individual United Way centers, particularly regarding operational and back-office functions such as finance, human resources, pledge processing, and communications. With greater demand for services and contracted resources, conversations began about how a group of United Ways could be structured differently. The seven organizations shared a similar goal: to positively impact lives by focusing on meeting community outcomes in the areas of education, health, and income in the Delaware Valley. The organizations were also in close geographic proximity. Thus in January 2010, together with assistance from an outside consultant, local United Ways began to explore what a more strategic partnership—including a merger—might look like. In September 2010, volunteers from nine local United Ways were brought into the discussion. These United Ways recognized the value of tackling regional education, health, and income through a united effort. Not only did the organizations at the table examine their commonalities, they also came to value each other's ideas and frames of reference. Often, agencies underestimate the importance of this process (Kirkpatrick, 2007), but it was crucial in this case because it permitted all agencies to conclude that merging was a good idea because of mission alignment rather than for any ulterior reasons such as financial instability.

As possibilities of a merger grew, two of the eleven United Ways that participated in the design process decided they were not ready to enter into a letter of intent (LOI) as of January 31, 2012. Of the nine United Ways that did enter into an LOI, seven ultimately signed the final plan and merger agreement; the remaining two decided it was not the right time for their communities, though each had different reasons. Figure 9.2 displays the service area map of the new UWGPSNJ.

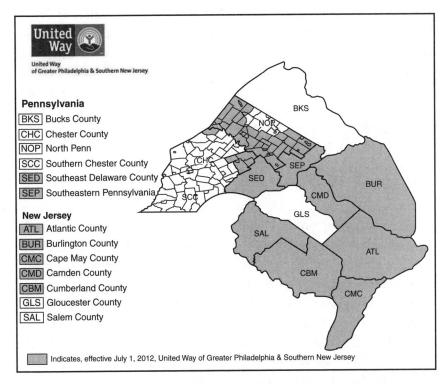

FIGURE 9.2   UWGPSNJ current service area map.

The Regional Design Team

For more than a year, the United Way design team chaired by Mindy Holman (president and CEO of Holman Automotive and board member of the former United Way of Camden County) and John Emge (executive director of the former United Way of Atlantic County), met bimonthly and then monthly to have what started as exploratory discussions about regionalization that ultimately led to the merger. In addition to the cochairs previously listed, the design team comprised the chief professional officer and two board members from each participating United Way. Team members were able to come together in a cohesive way to discuss processes, getting to know each other and establishing trust along the way, so that in the end everyone left at the table agreed to the merger for the right reasons. As Mindy stated, "It wasn't about what anyone was giving up but it was about what we were going to gain by coming together. It was a long process and sometimes a hard process, but it was a great process" (M. Holman, personal communication, July 10, 2012). In addition, staff and volunteers participated on subcommittees including the communications, community engagement, finance, governance, human resource, and information technology groups.

The design team's value proposition was, "To recommend the best alignment of financial and personnel resources for the most consistent, competitively priced donor experience to generate and leverage the greatest impact on local community needs that improves lives throughout the Greater Philadelphia market" (J. Michal [president and CEO, UWGPSNJ], personal communication, July 12, 2012).

Through the design team governance subcommittee, staff and volunteers from representative United Ways proposed a new governance structure that consisted of an overarching regional board comprising representatives from each of the local United Way boards and communities. In addition, each local United Way would continue to have a local operating board responsible for overseeing the local work such as local fundraising, community outreach, and volunteer engagement.

As the agency moved toward a formal merger agreement, the regional design team (comprising representatives from all United Ways at the table) addressed specific questions and concerns from each local community. The team had members from each local United Way board, allowing each to represent the needs of its local constituents. Then each committee's group members would report back to the local community boards to discuss and address questions. This became an iterative process; addressing local community needs was integral to the process as the local boards ultimately voted on whether or not they wanted to become a part of the merger.

The Official Agreement

Nonprofit mergers must take legal steps to form a single agency (Dewey & Kaye, 2007). With pro bono legal help representing each of the local United Ways (with Dechert LLP as the pro bono lead), the design team put together a nonbinding LOI that outlined all of the issues and concerns that needed to be addressed if a plan and merger agreement were to be successfully executed by the end of April. Nine United Ways signed the LOI on January 31, 2012, and worked diligently through the functional, volunteer-led subcommittees to address each issue with a goal of signing the agreement on April 30, 2012. Seven United Ways signed the formal plan and merger agreement and officially became UWGPSNJ on July 1, 2012.

NEXT STEPS

The seven United Ways have merged legally and are actively engaged in this new and exciting challenge to become an integrated and collectively stronger regional organization. At the outset, back-office departments such as information technology and pledge processing were combined, strengthened, and delivered consistently across United Ways. At the same time, UWGPSNJ continues the transition by defining and identifying strategies to further its community work. Organizationally, the new United Way has developed a strategic executive team, and with its new direction, the leadership is evaluating current work and the strategic vision to answer questions including: How is a regional campaign and community impact agenda best structured to leverage our collective strength and consistently deliver strong results throughout the region while honoring local needs, differences, and relationships? What synergies can be capitalized on? Throughout the design process, each United Way, regardless of size, demonstrated its inherent strengths and shared its best practices. To make the most of this merger, the integrated organization needs to continue to leverage its collective strength while supporting each local community to jointly address its challenges in the context of an increasingly complex landscape.

Overcoming Challenges

One of the biggest challenges to the merger, yet the key to its success, was developing trust. In the beginning, the United Ways were not sure what they were going to lose by coming together. Yet as they worked collectively over the course of 2 years, they realized that it was not about what anyone was giving up but rather what everyone was going to gain by coming together.

Celebrating Successes

Throughout the regional design team process, many communities welcomed the idea of a merger and were extremely involved at the local level. The design team was dedicated to discussing all facets of the merger through an engaged, thoughtful, and deliberate process. Design team members engaged their local boards and advocated for the merger, in the end resulting in a successful outcome.

Joining back-office functions while also capitalizing on each agency's unique strengths will allow the regional organization to fundamentally grow. From the outset, the back-office functions were consolidated, creating a more efficient system with a lower overall administrative rate than those of many of the former United Ways. Individuals with expertise in different areas, such as planned giving, would be expanding and targeting donors throughout the region, providing a seamless United Way brand experience both where donors work and where they live. In the long term, UWGPSNJ expects that this leaner, more strategic agency will be able to attract additional funding and volunteers, expanding its reach to a broader region and ultimately having a greater impact on community transformation.

MERGERS IN PERSPECTIVE

Nonprofit mergers provide a variety of benefits including the opportunity for expanded social impact. As Leslie Crutchfield and Heather Grant describe in *Forces for Good*, one characteristic of a high-impact nonprofit agency is adaptation (Crutchfield & Grant, 2008). Identifying external environmental road signs (such as shifts in the market, political landscape, or population) and meeting these through internal changes, such as a merger, increases the opportunity for broader organizational impact. The United Ways noted the commonality in their shift toward funding programs that addressed education, health, and income and saw this as a chance to provide a common donor experience. In addition, creating new programs and processes to address new opportunities through experimentation and innovation is critical. Through the merger, UWGPSNJ worked on increasing internal efficiency through process innovation. Lastly, high-impact nonprofits modify their plans and programs to expand performance. Through the merger, United Way was using the best practices of the region and the community to inform program development and better serve the community at large. Figure 9.3 graphically displays the adaptation cycle recommended by Crutchfield and Grant.

CONCLUSION

The creation of UWGPSNJ promises to improve outcomes, expand impact, and increase donor communication. The former United Way of Southeastern Pennsylvania's rigorous performance metrics for granting general operating and programmatic support will be used in collaboration with each local United Way's best practices as the basis for a consistent and strengthened investment framework for all local communities moving forward, ensuring consistency and furthering the impact of each dollar donated to UWGPSNJ. Joining forces will also increase impact in the region by collaboratively working to expand

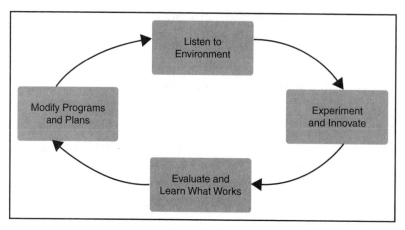

FIGURE 9.3 The cycle of adaptation.
Source: Cructchfield & Grant (2008).

high-quality education, increasing access to health care and promoting self-sufficiency. Lastly, the merger will create a seamless donor experience both at home and in the workplace. As John Emge stated, "A dollar donated will now make a footprint from Pottstown to Cape May" (J. Emge, personal communication, July 10, 2012). Finally, through the merger, United Way will have a greater voice in raising community awareness around the areas of income, health, and education disparities both at the local and state level.

CONTRIBUTING INTERVIEWS

Jill Michal, president and CEO, UWGPSNJ, and former president and CEO of United Way of Southeastern Pennsylvania; Mindy Holman, president of Holman Automotive Group, UWGPSNJ board member, chair of UWGPSNJ nominating and board development subcommittee and design team cochair, and former president and member of the board of United Way of Camden County; John Emge, executive director of UWGPSNJ in Atlantic and Cape May counties and design team cochair and former executive director of United Way of Atlantic County; Sara McCullough, senior director of regional integration at UWGPSNJ and former director of United Ways of the Delaware Valley.

AUTHOR'S NOTE

In preparation for this section of the chapter, the author interviewed four key local United Way leaders. The author heard a consistent message across the interviews, including a strong emphasis on trust building and a level-playing-field approach embraced by all leaders and members of the design team. The author's interview with Jill Michal aligned with that message. As the representative of the largest United Way in the design team process, Jill played a significant role in building an open and honest approach, establishing trust, and creating a space for everyone to have an equal voice regardless of the size of the United Way. As a longtime United Way volunteer from a smaller United Way in Southern New Jersey, Mindy Holman was also central in creating trust among United Way volunteers. Her approachable, even-keeled style allowed people to know they were heard while simultaneously driving the process forward. On the professional staff side, John Emge's commitment to local community presence and local relationships was a common goal among other professional staff members and was vital throughout the merger process. His knowledge, experience, and forward-thinking approach helped him and the other chief professional officers build trust at the local board and staff level. At the regional staff level, Sara McCullough's relationships and history with local United Ways ensured continuity and consistency across the design team, the consultant group, and volunteer and staff leadership, which was helpful in the trust-building and integration processes as well as the continued success of the merged organization.

THE ONONDAGA PASTORAL COUNSELING CENTER MENTAL HEALTH CLINIC: AN EMERGENCY MERGER OF TWO NONPROFIT ENTITIES IN SYRACUSE, NEW YORK

Carl M. Coyle

The Onondaga Pastoral Counseling Center (OPCC) was a long-standing mental health outpatient clinic with a nearly 40-year history of serving the community. Its risk of imminent failure was the result of poor strategic planning, adherence to a mission that was no longer viable or practical, and failure to act on emerging system changes in the behavioral health arena. In reality, this was a rescue as opposed to a merger. The clinic was so financially jeopardized that the situation required regulators to step in with interim financing while the legal issues were considered, because this was neither a formal merger, a stock sale, nor the assumption of a license.

BACKGROUND

Liberty Resources, Inc. (LRI) is a 501(c)(3) nonprofit corporately headquartered in Syracuse, New York. Liberty operates a wide array of behavioral health services across New York State (NYS) and Texas, and formerly in Florida. It also holds licenses to operate in Ohio and Pennsylvania and plans to strategically enter those states as well. LRI manages five primary service areas: Behavioral health, intellectual disabilities, child welfare, early intervention, and integrated primary care in its outpatient mental health clinics.

Founded in 1979 as a provider of community residence programs for mentally ill (MI) clients, LRI has grown from $500,000 in annual revenue to nearly $50 million. During that time, it expanded its scope and breadth of services by providing over 90 discrete programs that serve over 12,000 individuals annually. Specific treatment services include both residential and community-based nonresidential programs across NYS and Texas. The populations served are both adolescents and adults in all domains and include subpopulation care services such as juvenile justice, substance abuse and recovery, HIV/AIDS, foster care, school-based prevention programs, outpatient clinics, day habilitation, and others.

As referenced in earlier chapters, much of this growth has been organic. However, over time LRI has embraced the notion of both organic and strategic partnerships in order to attain scale and sustainability. With respect to mergers, partnerships, or affiliations, we ask ourselves three primary questions: Is there a community need and, if we are talking about an existing program, is it for services that are critical to the community? Can we operate the program with high-quality outcomes? Will it detract from the operating quality of our other programs? If the answers are positive to the first two and negative to the last, we will move forward to the due diligence phase. In partnerships and affiliations, this takes on a different approach as opposed to full-on mergers and rescues, as illustrated below. Similar to PHMC's methodological approach, nondisclosure agreements and formal due diligence are key components of the LRI process. It is noteworthy that much of our activity in M&A has concerned itself with rescues as opposed to *planful* mergers. In our experience, very few organizations are willing to contemplate merging for mutual gain, increasing scale and efficiency, or achieving greater mission impact. Too often, the notion of merging is seen as a threat to an agency's mission, as illustrated by the case study with OPCC below.

Very recently, in addition to the PPACA, a new element of health and behavioral health policy at the federal level has emerged. The Centers for Medicaid and Medicare has initiated pilot projects in several states including Texas, New York, New Jersey, Kansas, California, and Massachusetts for system changes related to both federal and state Medicaid and Medicare expenditures. Known as the Delivery System Reform Incentive Program (DSRIP), these major public policy initiatives focus on high-need/high-demand resource consumers. The services that are targeted most often are for chronic disease, mental health, and substance abuse. Increasingly, the sociological phenomenon of the aging baby boomer population as both Medicare and dual-eligible (Medicaid and Medicare) beneficiaries will consume a greater portion of health care dollars and the gross domestic product (GDP).

"Bending the curve" has become common in the lexicon of state and federal public policy. These policies, along with Balancing Incentive Program plans, amount to a redistribution of public dollars targeted toward high-need, high-use populations. How does this relate to affiliations, mergers, and partnerships? New and nontraditional affiliations are being forged between traditional human service nonprofit community agencies and hospitals and long-term-care entities. Forming alliances and strategic partnerships, these new delivery "systems" will thrive by achieving incentive financing based on outcomes. Clearly, there will be consolidation in the behavioral health and health care fields as dollars become more restricted and based on outcomes. The need for M&A, and for partnerships and affiliations, will increasingly become evident, with a distinct preference for organizational scale and broad geography for efficiencies of operation. Those community-based nonprofits that hold onto traditional methods of doing business and do not seek to form mergers, or even sound alliances, will find it increasingly difficult to survive.

The following illustrations of OPCC as a mental health provider and Cortland Community Reentry Program (CCRP; see section later in this chapter) for traumatic brain injury are leading indicators of this new reality. Over the years, LRI has conducted nearly 10 mergers or rescues. Some were planned, but most were not. At the time of publication, LRI was assuming another failed children's mental health clinic in Rochester, New York, and other mergers are being contemplated.

OPCC—RESCUE OF A FAILING NOT-FOR-PROFIT

Organizational History

OPCC was a nonprofit mental health center established in the mid-1960s with support from Dr. Norman Vincent Peale. The vision was to establish a pastoral counseling program based on Dr. Peale's concepts from the American Foundation of Religion and Psychiatry in New York City. The counseling program would have a distinct approach founded on theological counseling and training of clergy to provide counseling to individuals and families in Syracuse, New York. Its particular focus was to establish a center where clergy of various faith backgrounds could be trained in counseling with a particular treatment focus based on their religious beliefs. The founding board recognized that many people of faith seek counseling from their clergy as opposed to private mental health practitioners, particularly with regard to marriage and family counseling.

Established as a private, albeit nonprofit, center in an Episcopal church that was centrally located in Syracuse, OPCC accepted third-party insurance and established a sliding scale fee using both licensed and nonlicensed practitioners. Licensed practitioners were able to bill commercial insurance, and sliding fee scales allowed for the uninsured to be treated. The sliding scale also allowed nonlicensed clergy to counsel clients when insurance was not available. The first executive director was a licensed psychologist and minister and was therefore properly credentialed to facilitate training for the clergy.

Over the ensuing years, the center gained a reputation for clinical excellence and a willingness to treat people who did not necessarily seek treatment with a particular religious belief or desire for faith-based counseling. Beyond providing faith-based training, clergy were able to counsel in a center-based setting, benefiting from a clinically robust environment. This dynamic facilitated the expansion of OPCC's capacity and capabilities. By the late 1960s, the center had migrated toward group practice while retaining its pastoral counseling mission.

In the late 1960s, the board decided to seek status as a licensed mental health center under the NYS Department of Mental Health's regulatory requirements. This allowed for billing to Medicaid and Medicare and gave the center additional credibility. As a regulated clinic, OPCC came under a more rigorous set of operating standards but also became eligible for public funding and reimbursement as a licensed clinic. The center as a clinic was now required to appoint a medical director. Initially, psychiatric coverage was part-time, but as the number of people seeking treatment grew along with the number of treatment staff, the need for additional psychiatric coverage—particularly medication prescribing—began to expand. To a certain degree, the center was a victim of its own clinical success.

In the mid-to-late 1990s, as the mental health system began to change nationally related to managed care initiatives, OPCC found itself caught in the vortex of these system changes while struggling to meet its original mission of pastorally focused counseling. Client volume and a shift to the "public" client began to cause a strain on its finances. According to center staff at the time, the director was not particularly adept at managing the organization's finances. The cash balance of $400,000 was depleted, and the clinic declined into an operating deficit. Client caseloads continued to grow, to a peak in 2006 of over 800 active clients. However, vestiges of the "old way" of practicing remained. Many of the staff were part-time and performed as if it were still a group practice with a bias toward a pastoral mission. The training program for clergy became diluted, and fees for training clergy no longer sustained the cost of training.

In 2000, a new director was hired, and finances stabilized for a few years. However, the client demographic of predominantly Medicaid and Medicare beneficiaries, coupled with inadequate third-party insurance reimbursement, challenged the entity's financial viability. Because of flat reimbursement rates and changes in its payer mix, by 2002, the organization was again operating in a deficit.

The Merger Plan

In 2002, the executive director (ED) approached LRI and sought a merger. It was the assessment of the board and the ED that OPCC was not sufficiently diversified or of sufficient scale to weather the headwinds of system and reimbursement change. Meanwhile, LRI had grown from $19 million to over $28 million and continued to diversify its scope of services and geographic reach. Plans were in place to expand into other states as well.

As was typical with most mergers, the question of executive leadership became an issue. Much has been written on the fundamental economic differences in business drivers and motivation between the nonprofit and for-profit business sectors. Simply put, the economic benefit and resulting financial incentives to executives in the for-profit sector is not present for nonprofits. There is little (if any) financial gain for nonprofit executive leadership from mergers because of their inability to issue stock or other significant financial rewards for effecting the mergers. Thus, the critical question that quickly emerges in nonprofit mergers is, "Who will stay and who will lose their jobs as CEO?" As the reader will understand later, the question of executive leadership and control becomes a key element in the success of mergers. The attendant cultural integration issues that inevitably result from any merger, affiliation, or acquisition are significantly impacted by the question of executive leadership, particularly when the previous leadership is retained post-merger.

In this case, the CEO of OPCC was ready to retire, and thus the question of leadership control was mitigated. While the board was not in full agreement with the need for a merger, they allowed the exploration of the concept based on the organization's declining financial health and the executive director's planned retirement. The seeds of this less-than-focused strategy for organizational survival (and desire to thrive) impacted the outcome of this approach.

From early 2002 through early 2004, the executive teams examined their merger options. OPCC's clinical leadership and staff did not embrace the executive director's notion of the need for a merger. Much time and discussion were dedicated to continuing OPCC's pastoral care mission even though the center had essentially lost its vigor and its capacity to sustain this vision. Importantly, OPCC had effectively become a public outpatient clinic not unlike any other publicly funded program. The notion of pastoral care had become limited and no longer consistent with OPCC's current reality.

The protracted time and effort to examine the merger was acceptable to LRI because of its strategic desire to acquire a license for clinic services. NYS had had a moratorium on issuing any new licenses for over a decade. Barriers to care for LRI clients were a significant concern because of limited access, and it was believed that if LRI operated its own clinic, access and client care would be significantly improved across a spectrum of clinical needs (e.g., child and adolescent care, individuals with co-occurring disorders, and dually diagnosed populations). The protracted amount of time, nearly 2 years, proved to be a fundamental strategic error that caused the plan to merge to fail. As the due diligence discussions ensued, the boards were kept apprised, and the executive leadership of both entities began to reduce staff involvement because of both staffs' aversion to change. Despite assurances, OPCC staff feared that the larger nonprofit would "take over" the clinic and destroy its mission.

In mid-2004, both boards were sufficiently comfortable with the notion of a merger and were prepared to vote. Legal counsel was retained, and the respective boards went through the process of preparing for a legally binding vote. Because of the contentious nature of the decision on the part of the OPCC staff, great care was taken to ensure that the vote was legally binding. There were also lingering liabilities discovered during the due diligence phase that needed to be resolved. As such, both boards proceeded very cautiously.

In 2004, the respective boards of directors voted, and both affirmed a full merger. However, during the review of OPCC's bylaws, it was discovered that a quorum of the full board was required to take a legally binding action. When the board convened for the vote, a majority of members were present, voting unanimously, but the full board was not there. This delay required OPCC's board to take a second vote with all members present. That delay was fatal to the overall merger. Staff used the ensuing weeks to lobby the board to vote against the merger. Board members, several of whom were already ambivalent about the merger, listened to staff assurances that they would do what it took to reverse the financial loss. When the second vote was called, it failed to pass. Over two and a half years of time and effort resulted in failure.

The Saga Continues

In the meantime, LRI continued to expand and further its base of operations, becoming even more diverse and financially successful. It expanded into Florida in 2004 and had plans for entering Texas. Significant growth required the organization to purchase a second building for its programmatic and administrative activities because it had outgrown its current space. To quadruple the office space, an adjacent building was purchased in 2007 to accommodate LRI's continued organizational growth and development.

Meanwhile, OPCC continued to struggle. The former executive director retired, and an interim director was brought in to stabilize the center. In 2005, a permanent executive director was selected. The center attempted to stabilize itself, but it was not successful at implementing strategic plans to diversify or launch a planned giving campaign. Even under new leadership, OPCC could not generate a surplus, and its financial health continued to decline. By 2007, it was evident that in order to continue operations, OPCC would require an emergency cash infusion in order to stay open while it sought an organization to rescue it and assume its license. By this time, the organization was destitute and beyond salvage or repair. The state agreed to a one-time bridge loan of $300,000 to keep the center functioning that it would not be required to repay if a successor agency was found. Curiously, the board did not resurrect the previous merger discussions with LRI but instead chose to issue a request for proposals (RFP) for agencies interested in assuming its operating license. In some respects, OPCC wasted valuable time by following a competitive approach. The potential for a merger became the desperate need for a rescue.

Contextually, it is important at this juncture to understand the importance of the risk to the community if the center were to close. There were only six public clinics serving the metropolitan statistical area (MSA) of Syracuse with its approximately 450,000 residents. There is a state psychiatric center in Syracuse that serves adults as well as children and adolescents. In the late 1990s, it had refocused its emphasis to be less of an acute care psychiatric inpatient hospital because local hospitals had taken up the challenge of serving acute psychiatric care needs. Of the five remaining outpatient clinics located in Onondaga County, two were state run and had limited capacity and no ability or desire to expand. One was county operated, and with the economic stress on counties, it had no mandate to expand. This would have left one hospital-based outpatient clinic and one small clinic to meet the demand for the entire MSA if OPCC failed. The system had no capacity to rapidly absorb over 800 individuals, many of whom were chronically MI.

Two nonprofit agencies formally responded to the RFP, LRI and one other. In the end, the board selected LRI primarily because the center could no longer effectively operate in the church building where it began services in 1966. The church was forced to consider other tenant opportunities to pay the rent that OPCC could not, and the clinic received notice of eviction. In part because LRI was actively developing the new office building and had sufficient space to relocate the clinic, it was selected by the OPCC board to assume the operating license.

The time frame for actuating what had now become an emergency rescue was unrealistically short. Presentations to the board explaining the RFP response were held in August 2007, and the center estimated that it had sufficient cash (left over from the state's infusion) to operate through December of that year—otherwise it would close. Instead of conducting due diligence and careful planning in the planned strategic merger as before, the full effort—including NYS's transfer of the license—needed to be concluded within 4 months. Build-out for the clinic in the new space would take 10 months, and the lease with the church terminated in December 2007. Due diligence had to again be conducted because the lingering liabilities that had previously been discovered had worsened. In order to work around these, it was determined that there would be no license transfer, nor would there be a stock or asset sale or merger. LRI would file an emergency application with New York for a license, and OPCC would voluntarily surrender its license when LRI could begin operations. This would keep the liabilities discovered during due diligence from attaching to LRI. All due diligence, space planning, on-boarding of 45 staff members, case transfers, patient notifications, records transfers with consents, licensure, state certification, and system setup for billing and accounting had to be accomplished in less than 4 months.

On December 28, 2007, LRI was awarded an operating license by New York's Office of Mental Health. On January 2, 2008, LRI treated its first clients. Space in an existing building was converted and certified by the state, and half the clinical team moved into temporary offices while the new building was being renovated. The church agreed to extend a month-to-month lease because they were now receiving lease payments as they secured a new tenant for the space vacated by OPCC.

Construction costs, furnishings, and equipment came to over $1 million. Attention to detail for the new space paid off in terms of capacity building, functionality, and the quality of the environment. A significant increase in the number of counseling rooms was part of the vision for the new clinic, with capacity tripled to almost 50 therapy rooms. As part of the clinic's revitalization, capacity was increased to include group therapy, play therapy, family counseling rooms, and training facilities in the new space. An electronic medical record was implemented where OPCC had previously used paper charts. While all counseling rooms were insulated for confidentiality, white noise systems were installed along with new computers and office furnishing. A full-time medical director was hired, as were part-time psychiatrists who specialized in child, adolescent, and adult mental health, forensics, and substance abuse for patients with co-occurring disorders. The clinic was now much more robust, from its space to its treatment to its psychiatric capacities. In addition to the aforementioned improvements, there was also a significant investment in staff.

Staff had not received salary increases since 2005, so salaries were increased to market rates. Insurance coverage was brought level with that of other LRI staff members who enjoyed fully paid employer premiums.

OPCC's executive director and clinical leadership were retained because LRI did not have the staff capacity to undertake $3 million in services. This would have significant cultural integration ramifications over the ensuing months. Despite the considerable amount of time and effort, investments in staff compensation and benefits, staffing and physical plant improvements, and so on, the issue of cultural integration was a tremendous barrier in the initial phase of the rescue.

Much effort was expended on paying attention to differences in organizational culture and integration. The cultural divide, particularly on the part of the formerly OPCC staff, was a significant barrier. Absorbing the entire leadership team from the previous entity was a strategic error: What would change about the clinic's operation if all that was done was spending more money on staff salaries, equipment, and space without achieving a culture shift aimed at financial viability related to productivity? In fact, nothing was different. Staff remained allegiant to the previous executive director—all that had happened from their perspective was that a corporate sponsor had come in to underwrite the previous agency's poor business and practice management activities. A fundamental shift in organizational thinking and culture was needed.

An attempt was made to incentivize staff toward a culture of financial viability and sustainability by introducing performance bonuses that would be based on increased productivity and individual performance. Staff members who exceeded target utilization thresholds were awarded bonus checks above their base pay every 2 weeks. Interestingly, this had no effect on productivity or on moving toward a financially sustainable clinic practice; LRI simply spent more money on the staff members who were already exceeding utilization expectations. Those staff were exceeding expectations regardless of the bonus, and those who did not meet their targets were still receiving a full paycheck and better benefits. There was little incentive to change old habits.

Within 6 months, it was evident that there needed to be a culture shift to one that was aligned with LRI's culture of expectations. Accordingly, a wholesale change in the leadership structure was implemented. Both the previous executive director and the previous clinical director were dismissed. With new leadership in place, staff were subject to performance expectations and bonuses ceased. It would require a team effort to bring the overall clinic to profitability. Thus, a team structure around all clinical services was instituted, and clinical supervisors worked with individual therapists who were not meeting productivity standards. Staff who did not perform according to established standards either clinically or based on utilization were provided the opportunity to improve or they were terminated. Slowly, a culture of accountability and expectancy was created. This took a significant amount of organizational effort and patience, but it paid off. Within 3 years, the clinic had more than doubled its patient population to over 1,800 in active treatment. More importantly, the practice of "capture and hold"—keeping clients in therapy for 10, 15, or 20 years—was discontinued. The clinic now served more patients, and its unduplicated count increased from 800 to approximately 2,500 patients served annually.

These changes brought about a significant change in the staff's practices and pride. Coupled with reimbursement changes and better financial management, the clinic began to operate at a profit.

Today, the LRI clinic is the largest outpatient mental health clinic in central New York. Extension clinics have expanded to two additional counties, and the clinical staff has more than doubled. New therapies such as DBT and Suboxone treatment for individuals with co-occurring disorders are available. New strategic alliances with teaching hospitals and Syracuse University have infused new clinical capabilities and capacity.

Based on the success of the turnaround, in 2014, NYS awarded LRI a grant to establish primary care in the clinic setting. With the integration of behavioral health and primary care in one location, a more comprehensive treatment approach will be realized. The primary care clinic launched these services in the summer of 2014 and expects to scale services to over two-thirds of the clients served.

SUMMARY, OBSERVATIONS, AND LESSONS LEARNED

Many lessons were learned, and many strategies are being employed that differ from this case illustration as we continue to conduct mergers, acquisitions, affiliations, and rescues. Affiliations consume far too many leadership and administrative resources and are a strategy that LRI no longer pursues unless they are related to DSRIP activities, of which there are many. Provider associations in the era of increased managed care may prove an additional exception to this rule. With respect to the rescue of OPCC, there were both specific and global lessons learned—the most important was that the *integration of cultures is the most difficult aspect of any merger.*

Lessons Learned

- While *After the Merger,* listed as a resource, is an excellent guide to integration post-merger (or rescue), the amount of time and effort required after the legal transaction is complete cannot be underestimated. A significant investment of management's time should be expected. Staff charged with leading the new initiative should recognize the amount of time needed at the executive and senior leadership levels.
- Legal issues must be completely understood and resolved in concert with regulatory bodies in order to manage liabilities and risk. This due diligence is critical.
- Absorbing existing management generally results in ineffective integration and lessened potential for success. If the entity was not effective before, it probably will not be after the merger if the same management is retained.
- If the conceptual terms of a merger at the leadership and board levels cannot be resolved within 6 months, walk away—it is probably not going to happen.
- If the partnership was a rescue, do not expect any meaningful return on investment (ROI) for 3 to 5 years while the target is assimilated and "fixed."

RESOURCES

Bassi, L., Frauenheim, E., McMurrer, D., & Costello, L. (2011). *Good company: Business success in the worthiness era.* San Francisco, CA: Berrett-Koehler Publishers, Inc.

Pritchett, P. (2007). *After the merger: The authoritative guide for integration success.* New York, NY: McGraw-Hill.

CORTLAND COMMUNITY REENTRY PROGRAM, UPSTATE AND HUDSON VALLEY, NEW YORK

Carl M. Coyle

The assumption of a for-profit entity providing traumatic brain injury (TBI) and home care services that was at risk of ceasing operations.

The Cortland Community Reentry Program (CCRP) transitioned its TBI program under the sponsorship of LRI in 2011. As with the rescue of OPCC, assuming the failing program also required working with regulatory bodies to ensure service continuation until LRI could be licensed as a TBI provider. The situation had similar legal issues to those found with the OPCC rescue, which if conducted as a merger would have created a "successor and assigns" relationship. Trailing liabilities, legal entanglements, clinical records, and employee benefits each had to be considered in the process of this endeavor, with time of the essence (the transition was completed in 10 months) to avoid interrupting services.

However, the enterprise needed a significant infusion of cash and organizational resources in order to stabilize it. This included debt restructuring, costs associated with bringing the services into health and safety compliance, capital improvements, and employee benefits.

Several unknown risk elements also emerged that management did not disclose in the due diligence phase. Furthermore, the risk of a lawsuit from the previous operator also emerged, which could have had a significant financial impact on LRI had the suit been brought.

CONVERSION OF A FOR-PROFIT ENTERPRISE
TO NONPROFIT STATUS

The executive director of CCRP approached LRI in 2009 to discuss ways that the two organizations might collaborate. He identified concerns about the program's continued financial viability. Located in Cortland, New York, CCRP had also assumed responsibility for another TBI service provider downstate in Newburgh. Together, these programs represented the main service mix of the TBI enterprise.

As a long-standing business, CCRP was organizationally linked to a privately held system of long-term care nursing facilities that also admitted TBI patients. Within this corporate structure, CCRP's continuum of care operated structured day programs (rehabilitation) in Cortland and Newburgh as well as home care for individuals who could live semi-independently. The executive director indicated that as a system, CCRP had operated very profitably for over 20 years. The owner of the facility, who also owned other nursing homes throughout New York, had died. At the time, the legal status of the various business enterprises was unclear, but according to the executive director, CCRP began to deteriorate financially. Some of this was attributed to having shuttered the home care arm of the business, which had been profitable.

He reported that there were cash flow issues and that the program was operating at a significant loss. His concern and reasoning for seeking a merger emanated from the belief that the program was headed toward insolvency and would be closed.

While the corporate parent took the position that costs had to be cut and utilization increased (both of which were true), the executive director believed that not much more in the way of cost containment could be achieved. Staff had not received raises in some time, and there was no employer participation in health insurance premiums. Many of the staff went without health insurance because they could not afford it. Hourly wages were below market, and in some instances at minimum wage. With a diminished ability to recruit staff due to below-market compensation and benefits, increased utilization was a limited option. The executive director explained that his motivation for seeking a community-based nonprofit was that it would not have profit as a primary motive. He stated that he saw LRI as a well-run organization that was committed to quality and that perhaps had the financial resources to help fix the situation. The Liberty board considered the notion of committing to TBI services and another rescue but not as a takeover of the existing business or license. The OPCC experience had taught them that trailing liabilities invariably exist and that despite best efforts, they can never be fully determined. It was assessed that the best course of action would be to seek a new license and compete with the existing program. The leadership team was anxious to move to a community-based nonprofit provider and indicated that they would join LRI if it were granted an operating license by NYS. None of the leadership staff were under employment contracts, and therefore non-compete concerns were not a consideration.

Working with regulators, Liberty applied to the NYS Department of Health to become a TBI provider in 2010. Because of the complicated regulatory process, it took nearly a year to become approved. In the meantime, the bank holding the mortgage on the building CCRP occupied filed for foreclosure. Staff reported that health and safety issues had also emerged as a result of contracted services not being paid for, and it was becoming increasingly difficult to meet payroll.

In 2011, LRI was approved as a licensed TBI provider for the rehabilitation portion only. Home care services would be added later. It was assessed that assuming two locations and four program initiatives (rehabilitation, independent living skill training, case management, and private pay patients) was a sufficiently challenging task. Attempting to also launch the home care program, which required a separate state license, was determined to be too great a financial risk for the organization.

As the program sought space from which to provide services, it became clear that the simplest solution was to approach the owners of the current program site to see if a mutual compromise could be reached with regard to assuming the building and program obligations without purchasing the book of business. The leadership had already made it known to the corporate parent that they planned on leaving CCRP's employ and joining LRI. After a period of negotiation, it was agreed that the parent company would sell the program site to LRI. This in essence allowed the program to be subsumed under

LRI, with the parent walking away from the problems associated with the operation. In the end, all operations would be under LRI as the new corporate sponsor with existing management in place. While this relieved the parent corporation from the program's operating burdens, it was significant that the legal agreement and structure, as with OPCC, was not a stock or asset sale; LRI was a newly licensed provider that assumed the services.

Importantly, this served to insulate LRI from trailing liabilities and other risks. For example, CCRP had in the past undergone a Medicaid audit. Any findings under that audit would have been LRI's responsibility if the process had been a merger or asset or stock sale. This legal distinction ensured that any findings from the audit were not LRI's responsibility.

With the building secured from the previous owner, in the spring of 2011, LRI assumed operational responsibility for the TBI program. By the time negotiations for acquiring the building from the parent company and bank financing for the property were concluded, the program had further deteriorated financially. Clients left to choose other providers who were more stable, and the last of the home care clients were transitioned to other providers because the license had expired for that program. This left a program under greater financial stress than before. As with OPCC, there needed to be a significant infusion of cash and management time and effort. The previously known health and safety concerns needed resolution before the program could be certified as operational. New equipment had to be ordered and facilities had to be improved. The relatively new bus for transporting clients to community activities was inoperable and needed repair.

Compounding the costs for needed improvements just prior to opening the facility, the lower part of central New York from Cortland to the Pennsylvania border experienced a severe springtime flood. Homes were completely destroyed by floodwaters, and the state declared the region a disaster area eligible for federal relief. The new facility was not spared in this catastrophe. Fortunately, the building only suffered minor water damage, which required new carpeting, painting, and exterior repairs. The delay in commencing operations added to the financial strain already placed on the program. Staff were being paid, but very little billing could occur. The Newburgh program continued operations, but it was operating at a greater loss than the upstate program.

In the case of the TBI program (as opposed to with OPCC), the leadership team historically had a proven track record of quality services and financial success. According to the executive director, much of the financial decline could be linked to the parent corporation's financial challenges and, specific to the TBI program, the loss of the profitable home care program. As such, under LRI the strategic plan was to reinstate the home care division and grow back utilization by underwriting the program until it was financially viable. From the board's perspective, this was consistent with the organization's mission and served to sustain a much-needed, high-quality community service. It was also assessed that executive leadership was effective and did in fact operate with high-quality standards and effective financial performance, so long as the full service mix was in place. The loss of the profitable book of home care business was not attributable to the program per se. Accordingly, the leadership was retained to operate the program. Sadly, one simple decision on their part would prove to be the undoing of that decision and in the end forced that leadership to resign.

The on-boarding of staff went quite smoothly. Staff were happy to have their jobs without fear of layoffs or closure. Financial analysis indicated that bringing the staff up to market rates of pay was not immediately sustainable, but a significant commitment was made to pay 50% of insurance premiums immediately and to bring premiums fully on par with those of other LRI staff by the second year of operation. Cultural integration issues were more effectively addressed by building teams from both organizations to work on specific operational integration issues and to address programmatic barriers as they arose. Mentors were assigned to key staff, and all of the staff took great interest in making the new venture a success.

As the leadership decided who from the previous staff to offer employment, their thinking was not as discerning or critical as it should have been—all staff members were brought on board. In dealing with compensation for one particular staff member, it was explained that a raise was simply not feasible at this time. The organization needed to achieve a surplus before monies could be reinvested in salaries, and the commitment to pay for insurance premiums for all staff needed to be met; this alone was estimated at nearly $100,000. Later, this staff member became disgruntled and filed a complaint with NYS against the director and his deputy director alleging patient abuse.

When the state called to inform LRI that a complaint had been registered, they took the unusual position of conducting their own investigation into the matter. Unlike with other complaints or allegations the organization had received, the state refused to either elaborate on the charges or allow the agency to conduct its own investigation and report the findings to the state. NYS typically has an agency conduct its own internal investigation and always retains the right to come in after the fact to rereview the case if they do not feel the investigation was objective or thorough. This highly unusual stance, particularly from a new, albeit well-regarded, provider that had saved the program, was perplexing. Until the investigation was concluded, the state demanded that the leaders be placed on administrative leave. After nearly 10 weeks, the investigation was concluded.

The specific allegation and findings were not released. It was the state's ultimate and unilateral decision that the complaint was founded and that the leadership of the program "could have nothing to do with the program or any other program that derived its funding from Medicaid." LRI was free to employ them anywhere else in the agency but could not bill Medicaid for TBI or any other Medicaid-funded services they might oversee. LRI had no choice but to terminate the employment of the two leaders who had ultimately saved the program from closure. In a lamentable commentary, the director later said that the employee who filed the complaint had been difficult in the past and never should have been offered a position with the new program. His failure to critically analyze which staff should be on-boarded had cost him his job.

The former parent corporation's decision to focus on cutting overhead and increasing utilization was correct and necessary in order to bring the program to financial stability. Just as OPCC held onto its mission after it was no longer practical, staff were holding onto certain practices and costs just as they had when they were making a profit. They failed to critically analyze areas in which costs could be contained or reduced. Meals were prepared for clients by a cook, and staff benefited from free lunches as well, but there was no regulatory mandate for a meal program. Indeed, the entire goal of the day program was to rehabilitate clients with the intent of helping them achieve maximum independence. Staff should have been assisting with client rehabilitation in meal preparation. A psychiatrist was on staff, and this too was not a regulatory requirement. By conducting business as usual, the program was preventing itself from implementing needed measures that would have helped make it financially viable.

As with most mergers or acquisitions, it is anticipated that one outcome will be the consolidation of certain activities to result in increased operating efficiencies and associated reduced costs. While this is often true, this goal in and of itself can be limiting. The expanded capacity achieved through merger activity can often hold greater value without necessarily achieving operational efficiencies or cost reduction.

In this case, there were no operational efficiencies to be gained; in fact, additional staff and financial resources had to be brought to bear in order to stabilize the operation. The gains to be achieved were increased organizational capacity, broader geographic reach (future opportunities), business line diversification, and the potential to earn profits that could be used for other organizational needs (e.g., information technology infrastructure).

Today the program continues to serve clients in the Cortland and Newburgh locations. The home care component was brought back online in 2013. It has not scaled to its previous size; it started with only 6 beds, as opposed to the 60 it had managed when it was profitable. The Cortland location is highly profitable, but the Newburgh location continues to operate at a deficit along with the home care start-up. In late 2013, LRI added early intervention services throughout NYS including Newburgh in the Hudson Valley. It is hoped that synergies in that location will result in a financial turnaround for Newburgh.

COMMON THEMES AND LESSONS LEARNED

Cultural Integration Is Critical to Success

From these two case illustrations, several common themes and lessons can be drawn. Foremost, as research in the book *After the Integration* documents, many mergers fail not because of the inherent potential of the merger but because the combined enterprise fails to adequately address the issues of cultural integration post-merger. No two organizations are the same. All have their own unique cultures, and reconciling these differences is paramount if the coming together is to succeed and produce the intended benefits. Indeed, research shows that most mergers actually deconsolidate in the long run. The Daimler-Benz/Chrysler merger is a study in cultural integration failure.

Leadership must establish a clear mandate to address cultural differences post-merger. This is critical to the ongoing success of the newly structured organization, and is particularly true when previous management is retained. At the outset, the greatest initial impact will be achieved by addressing issues related to quality and employee morale. However, first everyone involved must ensure that all stakeholders are aligned with the ultimate goal.

Leadership Change Is to Be Expected

Absorbing existing management usually results in ineffective integration and lessened potential for success. In LRI's experience, assuming existing management rarely works, particularly if the merger is in fact the rescue of a distressed entity. For whatever reason, if management was failing previously, it will likely be ineffectual under the merged scenario. Often this failure of leadership is blamed on lack of financial resources or on the organization's external limitations, such as constraining policy issues or reduced salaries and benefits. These often mask underlying problems associated with current leadership. It is the leader's responsibility (and the board's) to *anticipate* change and manage toward a solution that is reasonable for the organization. This can take many forms, such as identifying the need to merge *before* the changes occur, while the organization is healthy. In the above case illustrations, a significant amount of time, management energy, and money would have been saved had the entities sought merger partners while they were viable. Increasingly in the nonprofit sector, scale will be a critical factor in organizational sustainability. Attempting to be a niche player no matter how high the quality is a difficult and perhaps unsustainable approach in an increasingly complex environment.

A caveat to this is if the acquiring organization does not have the management depth or programmatic or technical experience; in that case, assuming existing management *may* make sense, but only after careful analysis. Too often, it is easy to succumb to "doing the deal" for the deal's sake, at the risk of assuming existing management shortcomings. Hiring new, experienced talent in these cases makes better sense and increases the odds for long-term success.

Manage Risk—Due Diligence Is an Absolute Requirement

Government's push for consolidation in the nonprofit sector is expected but not supported. Rarely (if ever) does government provide financial incentive for nonprofits to merge while they are still healthy. All too often, this reality results in government's stepping in after the fact, when an organization is in jeopardy. However, regulatory approval is invariably required because nonprofits cannot dissolve or merge without court approval. Allowing for this process must always be taken into account.

There are many excellent templates for the due diligence process. In order to manage the risks associated with both known and unknown trailing liabilities, there must be ample time for due diligence. The process should not be rushed to a point where steps are skipped. Yet due diligence cannot completely ensure that all risks are known or quantified. There will always be surprises. The "full" story is never fully known or told.

In this context, it should be assumed that it will take more management time, money, and organizational resources to conduct adequate due diligence than expected. And once the process is completed, the issues of cost, time, and management attention do not go away. It can take years to fix the issues at hand and see a ROI. One executive who has conducted several successful mergers with healthy organizations on a national level stated that "it always costs you more, takes longer, and the ROI both financially and organizationally is usually a minimum of 5 years."

Provisions for adjusting scenarios when financial expectations do not materialize must be considered in advance. Often costs are not the issue because these can be controlled, but revenue projections invariably fluctuate, often for the worse. ROI should not be expected before 3 to 5 years.

Know When to Walk Away

Understanding when the deal makes no sense and determining absolutes for when to walk away are critical. The contemporary thinking is that if the deal cannot be conceptually agreed to and analyzed within six months, both parties should walk away. In this context, understanding mutual gain is a key component of any merger consideration. Timing can be everything. Ensure that you are seizing the "right" opportunity. If you proceed, recognize that sunk costs are a part of any organizational coming together.

One Final Thought

Risk is rewarded through tenacity, hard work, and an unwavering commitment to quality. No two mergers are alike, but there are common threads of process and needs. Understanding the reasons for a merger, following the process, paying attention to culture integration, and understanding the primary goal are central to any successful merger endeavor.

FUTURES FORWARD: THE MERGER OF PHILADELPHIA FUTURES AND WHITE–WILLIAMS SCHOLARS

Joan C. Mazzotti

Two organizations. Two offices. Two staffs. Two histories. One purpose: to help Philadelphia's low-income, high-achieving high school students reach their dream of college and careers.

While many in the community viewed White–Williams Scholars and Philadelphia Futures as two well-established, effective nonprofits doing good work, we were, in fact, competitors. We were competing for attention in the schools, recognition for our work, and decreasing charitable dollars.

On July 1, 2011, White–Williams Scholars and Philadelphia Futures merged. Today we are known as Philadelphia Futures: A Union of White–Williams Scholars and Philadelphia Futures.

An Internet search for articles about nonprofit mergers yields many descriptions and analyses of failed mergers. But the merger of Philadelphia Futures and White–Williams Scholars defied the odds. In just 14 months, we went from the first exploratory conversations between members of the two boards to successfully closing the transaction. It has been an exciting journey.

Two Rich Legacies

Although the missions of Philadelphia Futures and White–Williams Scholars were almost identical, our service delivery models were very different.

White–Williams Scholars is one of the oldest public charities in the United States, with more than 200 years of service to the youth of Philadelphia. It has a long and highly regarded reputation of providing low-income students with the financial resources necessary to support their academic goals while they are in high school. In 2005, White–Williams Scholars made the decision to expand the scope of its services and launched College Connection, which added academic support and college guidance to augment the financial stipends provided to students. Since 1995, White–Williams Scholars has also administered the Charles E. Ellis Trust for Girls, which annually distributes more than $1.2 million to support educational and personal development opportunities for low-income girls living in single-parent households.

Since 1989, Philadelphia Futures has been driven by the belief that children raised in urban poverty can transform their lives through the power of education. Philadelphia Futures' centerpiece college access and success program, Sponsor-A-Scholar, has a more than 20-year record of supporting low-income Philadelphia students on the journey to—and through—college. Unique among college access programs, Philadelphia Futures delivers services to students beginning in ninth grade and continuing through college completion. During high school, we provide students with deep, intensive, and long-term services, including academic enrichment, college guidance, ongoing staff support, and one-on-one mentoring. Students also receive $6,000 for college-related expenses, and staff support continues throughout college.

Philadelphia Futures has also developed programs and services aimed at increasing college access and success for a broad range of students including (a) collaborating with other organizations to manage and administer scholarship and awards programs and (b) annually publishing and distributing *Step Up to College: Philadelphia's Guide to the College Preparation, Application, Admissions and Financial Aid Processes.*

Prior to the merger, White–Williams Scholars had 13 employees and an annual budget of $1.6 million; Philadelphia Futures had 17 employees and an annual budget of $1.9 million.

THE RATIONALE FOR THE MERGER

Because both organizations came to the transaction from a position of strength, ours was a merger of mission and purpose rather than economic necessity.

The vision for the merger was about growth and impact as well as leveraging resources and expertise. Both organizations wanted to serve more students and increase the depth of the services provided. The two boards of directors believed that a merger was a far more effective and cost-efficient way of achieving these goals than growing organically and independently would have been.

The boards also clearly recognized the increasing competition for decreasing philanthropic dollars. In addition, public funding was on the decline, which would directly or indirectly impact all nonprofit organizations. A merger would allow the organizations to not only share resources and expertise but also reduce "back of the house" costs. The vision was that, together, we would be the premier provider of college preparation and retention services for Philadelphia's students.

In terms of organizational leadership, the time was right for a merger: the longtime executive director of White–Williams Scholars had recently resigned her position, and the board was just beginning the search for a new director.

The Process

The process began with confidential, exploratory discussions among a very small number of directors from each organization. I participated in those discussions. Once the small group was comfortable that there was alignment in mission and approach, the boards were briefed.

The boards agreed unanimously to pursue more formal negotiations, and each appointed a transaction committee to represent them in the negotiations. Each party also hired counsel to draft the agreements and handle the legal work attendant to a merger. At this point, the parties engaged in a robust due diligence process because each party needed to fully understand the other's liabilities—once the transaction closed there would be no recourse.

The next step was to reach agreement on the key business terms. It was critically important to both boards that the negotiations continue to be confidential. We wanted to ensure a meeting of the minds on the key business points before the potential merger was introduced to our staffs, funders, and partners.

In our case, the fundamental business terms that needed to be negotiated and agreed upon included the following:

- *The organization's name.* We agreed that the name would be Philadelphia Futures. However, the great legacy of the White–Williams Scholars name was important to both parties, and we decided to feature it as a key component of the services we provide.
- *The corporate entity that would survive.* It was agreed that the White–Williams Scholars corporate entity would survive. This decision made the most sense from a legal perspective, and we all were honored to be a part of an organization with roots in the early 19th century.
- *The composition of the board.* We decided to simply merge the two boards. Other issues regarding board governance were deferred until the strategic planning process began, following the close of the merger.

Once we had agreed on the business terms, the parties executed a LOI, and a carefully orchestrated public announcement was made. We advised our staffs simultaneously and then we immediately began the process of outreach to key funders and partners and to hundreds of donors, volunteers, and other stakeholders.

Five months after the LOI was signed, the merger agreement was executed. The agreement set forth the legal framework for the transaction and the business terms. We jointly prepared for the closing of the transaction, which took place at midnight on July 1, 2011—the first day of the new fiscal year.

Although we did not hire a consultant to facilitate the merger, we did utilize three external resources:

- Each organization retained outside counsel to represent it in the process.
- We jointly hired a communications firm to help us share our message with both internal and external audiences.
- A HR specialist was brought on to support us during the transition.

Post-Merger Work

Immediately following the merger, there was much work to be done. While we simultaneously ran the newly merged organization and maintained the quality of our programming, our respective infrastructures had to be combined. Everything—our staffs, employee benefits, offices, computer systems, bank accounts, development efforts, and so on—had to be integrated. I often comment that immediately following the merger we were a bit like Noah's Ark: We had two of everything.

The biggest undertaking post-merger was the start of our comprehensive strategic planning process in September 2011. A new strategic plan was necessary to fully operationalize the merger and leverage its increased opportunities. During the 9-month process, we solicited the views of more than 150 stakeholders, and the plan was approved by the board in July 2012.

Our Plan for the Future

The strategic plan that emerged brought our new organization's priorities into sharp focus, and will inform operations and year-to-year planning as we move forward.

Our plan articulates the combined organization's mission, vision, guiding principles, and core values. Our goals are clearly identified, and how we will meet those goals is also clearly defined. The plan sets out a robust combination of proven and new programs and services to carry out the organization's objectives.

WHY OUR MERGER SUCCEEDED

It has been nearly 3 years since our transaction closed, and we have seen the vision for the merger realized. I believe the key factors in the merger's success were the efficiency and collaborative spirit with which both parties approached it, motivated by a shared goal of positioning Philadelphia's students for a bright future.

There is no doubt that the merger between White–Williams Scholars and Philadelphia Futures was a bold move by the organizations' leadership. While many nonprofit organizations consider such moves, the fear of change, institutional egos, and the inertia of one's own success often tend to be obstacles that cannot be overcome. The boards of White–Williams and Philadelphia Futures had the vision to see beyond potential barriers and challenges and possessed the courage to act. They recognized that the combined organization would be stronger than the sum of its parts.

TPFC: MERGING FOR THE FUTURE

James Moss

"Ultimately, a nonprofit sector that knows well how to collaborate will be far more effective in the pursuit of its public-spirited mission" (McLaughlin, 1998a, p. xxiii).

SUMMARY

In June 2008, two organizations that had each served Philadelphia's children for over 125 years merged to form a new nonprofit entity, Turning

Points for Children (TPFC). The two organizations, Philadelphia Society for Services to Children (PSSC) and Children's Aid Society of Pennsylvania (CASPA), had been in discussion for 2 years before the merger was finalized. Four years after the merger, the new organization is stronger programmatically and financially than the two independent organizations had been by themselves. More importantly, TPFC is now better positioned for continued growth with an ability to compete in the changing landscape created by Philadelphia's DHS and its attempt to streamline case management and promote accountability among service providers.

A CULTURE OF MERGING

"What's the problem? Why don't we get everybody in the room and talk about opportunities and ways to collaborate?" Questions like these led to an event sponsored by Philadelphia DHS to promote collaboration. A lunch meeting was convened, organizations held discussions, and then everyone went home and the subject was never brought up again. "That was my first lesson that this was a different world."

Mike Vogel, CEO of TPFC, came to the nonprofit world after a 20-year career at Johnson & Johnson. He joined PSSC in 2000 as the director of operations and programs. In 2004, he was appointed executive director and guided PSSC through the merger process along with his counterpart, Gail Ober, executive director of CASPA. While Mr. Vogel had no specific experience with mergers in the for-profit arena, he brought his corporate management experience to bear in navigating the nonprofit world and set about to look for a partner with whom to collaborate.

PSSC had previously attempted to merge with another nonprofit organization through a United Way grant. "I thought it was a great potential merger... This other organization didn't have an endowment, and so had to be really good at raising their full budget every year, and I thought to myself, 'That would be a great skill for us to add to what we were doing already,' because we weren't that good at it. I don't think we even had a development person at the time" (M. Vogel, personal communication, 2012).

Negotiations eventually fell through, but because the possibility of a merger had been explored, when the next opportunity came around, this time it was a success. While PSSC and CASPA had had no history of collaboration, Mr. Vogel's predecessor, Helen Dennis, mentioned that she used to talk with Ms. Ober over lunch about merging but that nothing more ever came of it. When Ms. Dennis retired and Mr. Vogel became CEO, he stated, "I don't remember if it was her [Ms. Ober] calling me or me calling her," but the discussions resumed and eventually turned into a serious effort focused on merging the two organizations.

In fact, one of the main reasons the Turning Points merger was successful was that both CEOs championed it. Early on they worked out how the management structure might look and what role each of them would play based on their respective strengths. This alleviated two of the common road blocks to merging. According to Tom McLaughlin, founder of the consulting firm McLaughlin & Associates and nonprofit merger expert, ego and economics (the two big Es) can be strong factors in individual staff and board member motivations, and can lead to active or passive efforts to sabotage negotiations (McLaughlin, 1998b). Because of the problem of conflicting motivations, organizations should use the absence of a CEO, for whatever reason, as an opportunity to explore merging (McLaughlin, 2004).

According to Mr. Vogel, "On paper we looked like a merger that could happen in a week. We had similar missions; both our agencies were old; we both had money.... There was a lot of synergy." McLaughlin says that the entities involved tend to forget that mergers take time, and argues that mergers and affiliations need to be built into the culture of organizations because "the integration process does take a long time." Therefore, you will be doing serial integrations if you are a large enough, complicated enough system. "Ultimately, you will build it into your structure, into your staffing, and into your culture and you will get good at this" (M. Vogel, personal communication, 2012).

While TPFC is not yet a large enough organization to process serial mergers on the scale suggested by Mr. McLaughlin, it does have a long history of mergers and affiliations dating back to 1898. At least seven different organizations have become part of the Turning Points pedigree (Figure 9.4). While neither PSSC nor CASPA has gone through a merger in the past 30 years, they are a part of each other's histories, along with their links to the 19th century. This shared identity helped

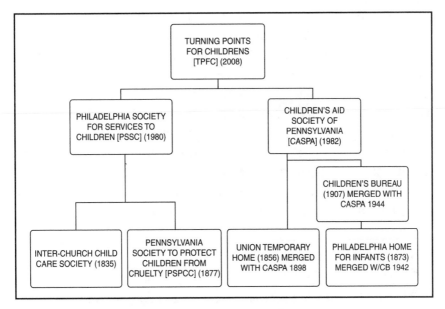

FIGURE 9.4   Organization merger history.

the leaders of the two merging organizations recognize each other as kindred entities with whom they can coexist.

PSCC was formed in 1980 as a merger of the Inter-Church Child Care Society (founded 1835) and the Pennsylvania Society to Protect Children from Cruelty (PSPCC). PSPCC was chartered in 1877 and was the eighth such group in the United States at that time. The building at 415 South 15th Street, current home of TPFC, had acted as PSPCC's headquarters from 1906 to 1980, when it became the headquarters for PSSC. The Inter-Church Child Care Society, formerly the Home Missionary Society, was founded in 1835 by members of the Methodist Episcopal Church as an evangelical group that, around 1854, "assumed the added task of placing poor dependent children in 'good Christian homes' in the country" (Clement, 1979, p. 137).

CASPA was organized in 1882 and provided services for Philadelphia's homeless and endangered children. During its long history, CASPA had absorbed two other organizations: the Union Temporary Home for Children (merged 1898) and the Children's Bureau (merged 1944). The Philadelphia Home for Infants (founded 1873) had previously merged with the Children's Bureau in 1942.

The Children's Bureau is an excellent example of the long history of collaboration among Philadelphia's nonprofits. Established in 1907 through a joint effort of PSPCC, CASPA, and The Adam and Maria Sarah Seybert Institution for Poor Boys and Girls of Philadelphia, the Children's Bureau acted as a joint shelter for the founding agencies as well as an information and education center for the more than 60 agencies in Philadelphia that received destitute children at that time (Gumbrecht 2003, p. 4). In 1908, a training program was developed to educate childcare social workers. This training program was the seed for what was to become the University of Pennsylvania's School of Social Policy and Practice (Lloyd, 2008, p. 4).

Institution Profile

In 2011, TPFC provided services to over 2,700 families and 5,300 children; Figure 9.5 gives an overview of TPFC's service and revenue profile. TPFC provides a variety of preventive programming and services for children and their families, working closely with DHS to help children in need through programs such as:

In-Home Protective Services—Providing parenting skills and protective capabilities for families in which children are at imminent risk of abuse or neglect

Families and Schools Together—A licensed, evidence-based program that works with schools and communities to provide parenting education and family support services

Time out for Teens and Tots—A parenting and support program for pregnant teens and teen mothers and their children

Family Finding—Reconnects youth in out-of-home care to family members with whom they have lost contact, to provide another network of support

Family Empowerment Services—In-home services that enhance parents' abilities to meet the basic and well-being needs of their children and prevent the onset of abuse and neglect

Kids N' Kin—Supports families of children being raised by a nonbiological parent (e.g., extended family member or family friend).

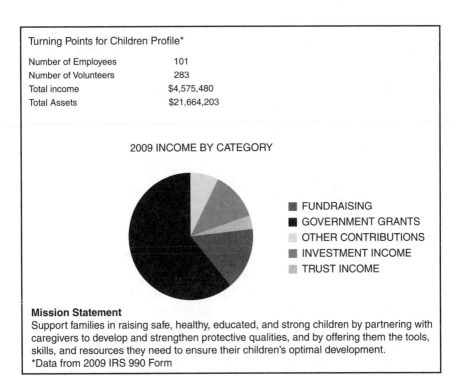

Turning Points for Children Profile*

Number of Employees	101
Number of Volunteers	283
Total income	$4,575,480
Total Assets	$21,664,203

2009 INCOME BY CATEGORY

■ FUNDRAISING
■ GOVERNMENT GRANTS
▨ OTHER CONTRIBUTIONS
■ INVESTMENT INCOME
▨ TRUST INCOME

Mission Statement
Support families in raising safe, healthy, educated, and strong children by partnering with caregivers to develop and strengthen protective qualities, and by offering them the tools, skills, and resources they need to ensure their children's optimal development.
*Data from 2009 IRS 990 Form

FIGURE 9.5   2009 Income by category.
Source: Data from 2009 IRS 990 form.

Nonprofits Coming Together

In 1998, Tom McLaughlin predicted that:

> The bulk of innovation today will take place not in programs and services, but in management. And the thrust of that innovation will be toward greater collaboration between nonprofit organizations and all others carrying out similar missions. What we call mergers and alliances are really just part of the innovation that the nonprofit sector must deliver over the next two or three decades. (McLaughlin, 1998a, p. xxii)

While the merging of nonprofit organizations has been on the rise since the 1990s, there are several different forms of partnerships that nonprofits can create. Nonprofit partnerships are typically divided into three categories: collaborations, alliances, and integrations (Kohm & La Piana, 2003, p. 5; Kohm, La Piana, & Gowdy,

2000). Collaborations occur when organizations share information or coordinate their efforts but each continues to act independently. Alliances take place when two or more organizations share programs or administration while also requiring shared decision making. Integrations involve a change in the corporate structure of the organizations, including mergers.

Motivations for partnerships include:

- perceived financial savings
- pressure from funders
- strengthening programming
- expanding mission
- taking advantage of a partner's area of expertise
- taking advantage of a partner's reputation

A successful nonprofit merger will cite a number of these factors as motivation to merge (Kohm et al., 2000). If the sole reason for a merger is to save an organization, it is too late (Gammal, 2007; McLaughlin, 1998a). For a merger to be effective, it needs to be considered before there are signs of trouble. When a healthy organization merges with a troubled one, all existing problems are also absorbed, which could threaten the stable organization. Gammal (2007, p. 48) cites the example of a $2 million health service provider that was pressured by funders to absorb a failing organization. The funders failed to follow through on promised financial support and caused the unexpected financial burden of renovation dollars, extra staff time, and lost revenue during renovations, which nearly bankrupted the formerly stable organization.

The best reasons to merge are mission and program. A 1999 survey of San Francisco Bay Area nonprofits found that, "Respondents entered into a strategic restructuring more often to improve the quality or range of what they do and the efficiency with which they do it than because of any immediate threats of closure or pressure from funders" (Kohm et al., 2000, p. 2).

There are two widespread assumptions that compel nonprofits to merge. The first misconception is that there are too many nonprofits in general. The second is that most of the ventures are too small and inefficient (La Piana, 2010, p. 28).

Philadelphia County (coterminous with the City of Philadelphia) and its surrounding four counties (Bucks, Chester, Delaware, and Montgomery) contain a total of 15,000 nonprofit organizations, 3,600 of which are public charities that serve individuals and households; 1,691 are categorized as human service organizations, with 658 in Philadelphia, including TFPC (The Philadelphia Foundation, 2010).

Fifteen thousand certainly sounds like a large number of organizations, but what does this mean? Too many for what? McLaughlin simply states that in many parts of the country, there are too many nonprofits and that "having an excessive number of nonprofit organizations actually weakens the collective power of the entire field…spending a disproportionate amount of resources worrying about how they are going to fund it, manage it, and perpetuate it" (McLaughlin, 1998a, p. xxii).

Public charities are defined as 501(c)(3) organizations, not including public foundations. In 2007, over one-third of the public charities in southeastern Pennsylvania were in the red; 9% had liabilities that exceeded their total net assets (The Philadelphia Foundation, 2010, p. 4). It could be argued that either there is just not enough available funding or the organizations in the red are not being managed properly. Either way, are these organizations collectively meeting their constituencies' needs? In most cases, when multiple organizations are providing the same services, it is not the redundancy of services that is the problem. In fact, this is usually an indicator that there is a greater need for services. It is the redundancy of infrastructure that is wasteful, not the duplication of services (La Piana, 2010, p. 30).

The second assumption, that most nonprofits are small and inefficient, is easier to demonstrate. The 1,691 human service organizations accounted for $1.8 billion in revenue (The Philadelphia Foundation, 2010, Philadelphia County, figure 2). Of these organizations, 39.6% were operating with deficits (Philadelphia County Data, figure 2; The Philadelphia Foundation, 2010). Generalizing across the larger category of nonprofits serving individuals and households in the 5-county area, the largest 10% of nonprofits accounted for more than 80% of the spending (The Philadelphia Foundation, 2010, p. 17).

Philadelphia's DHS Quarterly Contract Report in 2012 listed 227 child welfare and juvenile justice-related services contracts (three of which are with Turning Points) with a total of 169 organizations. While these contracts are not all for the same services, many do overlap, and Turning Points is, in essence, competing with 168 other organizations for DHS funding (City of Philadelphia, 2012a).

Of the nearly one million public charities in the country, 3.9% earned $10 million or more, accounting for 84.8% of total expenditures in the sector. Public charities that spent between $5 million and $10 million (including Turning Points) accounted for 2.6% of the organizations and 4.8% of the total expenditures. The vast majority of public charities, 73.9%, accounted for less than 3% of the total expenditures (Wing, Roeger, & Pollak, 2010).

In an environment in which multiple organizations provide the same services with competing infrastructures, it seems logical to bring these organizations together to eliminate redundancies and take advantage of efficiencies and economies of scale. However, in an attempt to save money during a merger, the new organization can find itself spending more:

> Despite conventional wisdom, mergers themselves do not generate revenue or reduce expenses. In the short term, they actually require new money for onetime transactional and integration costs. Even in the long term, the act of merging itself did not lead to substantial cost savings for the vast majority of the mergers my firm has facilitated. Merged nonprofits can roll together annual audits, combine insurance programs, and consolidate staffs and boards. But they are also bigger and more complex and require more and better management—a cost that often exceeds the savings from combined operations. (La Piana, 2010, pp. 30–31)

A survey conducted by The Stanford Project on the Evolution of Nonprofits in the San Francisco Bay Area reported that none of the merged organizations in its sample reduced its need for funding, because each merger was used to grow the organizations' activities, actually increasing the overall revenue requirements despite reducing the number of organizations (Stanford Graduate School of Business, 2005).

Economies of scale do not just apply to finances, however. A larger organization is able not only to negotiate better deals with suppliers but also to wield more clout by increasing its market share when dealing with foundations and government agencies. The more services an organization can provide in a community, the more indispensable it becomes. This allows for a stronger negotiating position to provide even more services, and ultimately permits it to grow.

Funders have been known to scale back funding to newly merged organizations, however (Gammal, 2007), so it is still up to individual managers to engage foundations and government officials effectively.

When nonprofits do merge, the most commonly reported benefits include increased services, increased administrative capacity and quality, and increased market share (Kohm et al., 2000, p. 2). Mike Vogel notes that while Turning Points has not seen obvious cost savings, they have increased their services and hired more employees. During DHS's recent restructuring, contractors for preventive services were cut from 40 to approximately 12. "And we were lucky enough to be one of that dozen. We grew in this time that others were shrinking, and this caused us to hire a lot of new people." Because human service is a labor-intensive field, Mr. Vogel estimates that 70% to 75% of Turning Points' costs are salary and benefits. "So we're buying more stationary, we're buying more cell phones, we're buying more computers. Is there cost savings? I think we're getting better deals now. We can negotiate better terms...but the overall expenses are more." Ultimately, however, as the organization has grown, so has its budget.

Cooperation Versus Competition

Competition in the for-profit world is viewed as not only healthy but also an integral and necessary part of capitalism. Competition weeds out companies that fail to provide quality goods and services at a competitive price. However, in the nonprofit arena, especially preventive human services, it is very difficult to assign impact to a particular program or service because of the multitude of variables involved. Therefore, ineffective programs can continue to persist despite their ineffectiveness because of contract failure, which occurs when those who receive goods or services are not the ones paying for them (Kohm & La Piana, 2003, pp. 12–13).

Yet nonprofits do compete for funding dollars from both public and private sources. Despite a reluctance in the nonprofit culture to admit to competition, it remains very real. Because of this fact, and in the face of the demonstrated advantages of organizations working together, nonprofit organizations must learn to be adept at both cooperation and competition, simultaneously (McLaughlin, 1998, pp. 80–81). Mergers and affiliations are one way that organizations are attempting to temper competition (Kohm et al., 2000, p. 2).

Funders direct monies to organizations that demonstrate efficiency or effectiveness. Sadly, often just providing the appearance of efficiency is enough. By merging, in addition to the other benefits, organizations can provide the appearance that they are serious about efficiency, making the case for even more donor dollars (Kohm & La Piana, 2003, pp. 14–15).

Navigating a Changing Landscape

Fourteen-year-old Danieal Kelly fell through the cracks in the DHS system. In 2006, Danieal was found dead of abuse and neglect, even though the family had reportedly received services for years. A grand jury indictment of nine individuals revealed a systematic failure of the DHS system to protect the young girl, who suffered from cerebral palsy. In response to Danieal's death and to others whom the DHS system failed to protect, a community oversight board (COB) was created to investigate the events that led to the tragedy and to provide recommendations for overhauling the system (McElroy, 2012).

Following in other state and government footsteps, the system overhaul in Philadelphia became known as Improving Outcomes for Children (IOC), which is aimed at streamlining the child welfare system by decentralizing direct case management services through a network of contracted Community Umbrella Agencies (CUAs). The program establishes "the foundation for a single case management system delivered by providers through the development of strong, geographically based, community-level partnerships" (City of Philadelphia, 2012b, p. 6). By clarifying the roles of DHS, providers, and subcontractors, IOC sought to eliminate redundancies while strengthening performance management and accountability structures. Ten CUAs were identified (and selected in 2012–2014), with geographic boundaries overlapping existing Philadelphia police districts.

This approach is based on the premise that positive outcomes are achieved through the use of child protection and child welfare services that are family-centered, community-based, culturally competent, integrated, timely, and accountable for results.

In order to achieve these positive results, particularly safety, permanency, and well-being for our children and youth, the system must promote new practices, service innovations, and true collaborative partnerships between public and private agencies and stakeholders in the communities served. (City of Philadelphia, 2012b, p. 4)

Prior to responding successfully to the two CUA proposals, TPFC in the spring of 2013 became a subsidiary corporation of the PHMC. The decision to join a large health and human service management agency like PHMC was to assure that Turning Points could successfully compete for the CUA business and have the infrastructure in place with the support of a parent corporation should it be needed.

In 2013, TPFC was one of the organizations that was selected to operate 2 of the 10 CUAs. Looking back, while PSSC and CASPA could not have predicted what the outcome of the COB would be, it was within this environment of change that they were negotiating to merge. Similarly, the affiliation with PHMC was also a leap of faith into the future. Kohm and La Piana (2003, p. 24) state that most of the organizations surveyed chose to consolidate "not because of what funders were doing at the time, but because of what they thought funders would do in the future." The CEOs and board members of PSSC and CASPA could not know what DHS would do in the future, but they knew the status quo was changing and that by merging, a new organization would be in a better position to compete.

Another benefit of the merger was that it enabled the new organization to weather the recent worldwide economic crises. A month after the merger was finalized, TPFC was in financial crisis mode. "This is where you could say we looked like geniuses," Mr. Vogel says. Either organization may have survived on its own, but even if they had, their endowments most likely would have been drained. Today, TPFC is a more than $30 million human service corporation, up from its $5 million revenue just after the merger.

Positioning for the Future

> When I first came, I looked around at the landscape, and I said, "Wow! we're really relatively small and insignificant." And we were. I think the work's really important. If what we do is as good as we say it is, then we need to find ways to deliver the work to more people, because god knows that there are more people out there than we serve. (M. Vogel, personal communication, 2012)

Preventive human services organizations generally depend largely on government funding; in 2009, nearly 75% of Turning Points' income was from government grants. Fundraising from private donations is time-consuming, and an uphill battle with the multitude of similar organizations in the area. There are fewer and fewer corporations based in Philadelphia, so that that funding stream is quickly diminishing. In general, foundation dollars are allocated for short periods of time so that foundations avoid becoming steady funding streams for organizations, which makes it difficult to build a financial strategy around foundation grants. What's left is government funding.

Mr. Vogel states, "In our work, part of my challenge is to make it hard for government to defund me." And so, in addition to having excellent programs and accountability, an organization has to do this on a scale that will be attractive to politicians. With the establishment of IOC, organizations will need to demonstrate that they can deliver services and manage accountability on a scale that Philadelphia human service groups have not been required to meet.

> If an organization depends on government funding, which more and more requires them to perform at a greater scale and level of accountability, how does an organization grow in order to create a greater programmatic footprint and justify additional funding? By merging.

By the end of 2012, four years after the Turning Points of Philadelphia merger, only two or three board members were left from the original boards of PSSC and CASPA. Between the process of the merger and the ensuing financial crises, many of the board members were fatigued. Partially due to the hiring boost from the expanded DHS contracts, only approximately 50% of the current staff was initially employed by either legacy organization. And while this was not part of anyone's plan, Mr. Vogel says that the influx of new staff really helped to change the culture of the new organization, reducing the "we used to do it this way" mentality and the resistance to new ideas.

Mr. Vogel believes that IOC spurred discussions among organizations that have explored the idea of partnering along the lines of creating a form of holding company, by which the various members could share the CUA contracts. But, he says, "The way the RFP was written you couldn't really afford to do that, and so you're left with doing it on your own, or merging or affiliating. No one seemed to be willing to want to merge. So we're back to doing it on our own and in partnership with our parent organization, PHMC. Or not doing it all and deciding what's best for us is being a subcontractor. Those seem to be the two options" (M. Vogel, personal communication, 2012).

Despite this apparent lack of enthusiasm on the part of other organizations, Thomas McLaughlin proffers, "I actually think that there may come a time when…the reaction which you would describe now is something like, 'Oh you had to merge your organization? Oh, you poor thing, what did you do wrong?' changes to, 'Oh, you mean you haven't tried an alliance? You haven't merged with another organization? What's wrong, why does no one want you?'" (personal communication, 2012).

Recently, Turning Points attempted to acquire a foster care agency. The negotiations failed because the agency chose to partner with another organization. But as long as TPFC continues to be open to the idea of growth through merger, it is only a matter of time before the right opportunity will present itself, and when it does, the organization will grow again. And it is that awareness of the environment and the willingness to both cooperate and compete that is the real innovation.

REFERENCES

Adams, C., Bartelt, D., Elesh, D., & Goldstein, I. (2008). *Restructuring the Philadelphia region: Metropolitan divisions and inequality*. Philadelphia, PA: Temple University Press.

American Psychiatric Association. (APA) (2000). *Diagnostic and statistical manual of mental disorders* (4th ed., text revision). Washington, DC: American Psychiatric Association.

Barnard, M., & McKeganey, N. (2004). The impact of parental problem drug use on children: What is the problem and what can be done to help? *Addiction, 99*(5), 552–559.

City of Philadelphia. (2012a). *Quarterly contract report: January 1, 2012 to March 31, 2012.* Retrieved from http://secure.phila.gov/ECONTRACT/ Documents/frmPDFWindow.as px?docid=95Q12N&ext=pdf&orig _name=Qrtly%20Rpt%204.1.12%20to%206.30.12_final.pdf

City of Philadelphia. (2012b). *Request for proposals for improving outcomes for children community umbrella agency for the city of Philadelphia.* Philadelphia, PA: City of Philadelphia Department of Human Services. Retrieved from http://dynamicsights.com/dhs/ioc/files/RFP_Final.pdf

Clement, P. F. (1979). Families and foster care: Philadelphia in the late nineteenth century. *Social Service Review, 53*(3), 406–420.

Crutchfield, L. R., & Grant, H. M. (2008). *Forces for good: The six practices of high-impact nonprofits.* San Francisco, CA: Jossey-Bass.

Dewey & Kaye. (2007). Nonprofit mergers: An assessment of nonprofits experiences with the merger process. *Tropman Reports, 6,* 11–19.

Gammal, D. L. (2007). Before you say "I do." *Stanford Social Innovation Review, 5*(3), 47–51. Retrieved from www.ssireview.org/articles/entry/ before_you_say_i_do

Gumbrecht, J. (2003). *Children's aid society of Philadelphia records.* In Collection 3026. The Historical Society of Pennsylvania. Retrieved from http:// hsp.org/site/default/files/legacy_files/migrated/findingaid3026chil-drensaid.pdf

Kirkpatrick, K. (2007). Go ahead—pop the question. *Stanford Social Innovation Review, 5*(3), 43–46.

Kohm, A., & La Piana, D. (2003). *Strategic restructuring for nonprofit organizations: Mergers, integrations, and alliances.* Westport, CT: Praeger.

Kohm, A., La Piana, D., & Gowdy, H. (2000). *Strategic restructuring: Findings from a study of integrations and alliances among nonprofit social service and cultural organizations in the United States.* Chicago, IL: University of Chicago Press.

La Piana, D. (2010). Merging wisely. *Stanford Social Innovation Review, 8*(3), 23–25.

Linehan, M. (1994). *Cognitive-behavioral treatment of borderline personality disorder.* New York, NY: The Guilford Press.

Lloyd, M. F. (2008). *A centennial history of the School of Social Policy and Practice.* Philadelphia, PA. Retrieved from http://repository.upenn.edu/ cgi/viewcontent.cgi?article=1000&context=centennial

McElroy, R. (2012, February). Innovation at the Philadelphia Department of Human Services (DHS): Improving Outcomes for Children. *Philadelphia Social Innovations Journal*. Retrieved February, 2012 from www.philasocialinnovations.org/site/index.php?option=com_con tent&view=article&id=406:innovation-at-the-philadelphia-depart ment-of-human-services-dhs-improving-outcomes-for-children- by-increasing-accountability-and-strengthening-community- partnerships&catid=21:featured-social-innovations&Itemid=35

McLaughlin, T. A. (1998a). *Nonprofit mergers and alliances: A strategic planning guide*. New York, NY: John Wiley & Sons, Inc.

McLaughlin, T. A. (1998b). Why Mergers Fail: Here's What to Do About It. *The Nonprofit Times*.

McLaughlin, T. A. (2004). Don't replace, merge: An open letter to board members. *The Nonprofit Times, 18*(23), 1–2.

The Philadelphia Foundation. (2010). *Nonprofit study*. Philadelphia, PA. Retrieved from www.philafound.org/Portals/0/Uploads/Documents/ Public/TPFNonprofitStudy.pdf

SAMHSA report finds 6 million children live with addicted parents. (2003). *Alcoholism & Drug Abuse Weekly, 15*(22), 5.

Stanford Graduate School of Business. (2005). *Managing through challenges: A profile of San Francisco Bay Area Nonprofits*. Stanford, CA: D. L. Gammal, C. Simard, H. Hwang, & W. W. Powell.

Wing, K. T., Roeger, K. L., & Pollak, T. H. (2010). *The nonprofit sector in brief: Public charities, giving, and volunteering, 2010*. Washington, DC: Urban Institute. Retrieved from www.urban.org/UploadedPDF/412209- nonprof-public-charities.pdf

10

Strategies, Tips, and
Legal Partnership Documents

EDITORS' OVERVIEW

By now, *Partnerships for Health and Human Service Nonprofits: From Collaborations to Mergers* has: presented an overview of strategic partnerships in the nonprofit sector; shared strategies for success; discussed some of the challenges to and dispelled myths about these partnerships; and presented case studies of both successful and not-so-successful partnership efforts. As has been emphasized, any partnership attempt is more likely to succeed with a thorough due diligence process on the part of all parties/organizations, and this chapter provides samples of some of the documents you can expect to complete during a partnership process, as well as checklists and other best practices documents to guide you. Although the book's case studies are based mainly in the Philadelphia area, these documents or variations on them should be applicable in any location.

Mutual Confidentiality Agreement

Prior to obtaining any documentation from another nonprofit corporation, each corporation should sign a confidentiality and nondisclosure agreement to frame the specific limits and uses of the confidential information that each party shares with the other.

Affiliation Feasibility Assessment

Public Health Management Corporation uses this information to initially analyze the viability of any form of merger, collaboration, or partnership with another nonprofit corporation.

Due Diligence Request List

No matter the form of partnership, collaboration, merger, or acquisition between corporations, a careful review of the legal risks and statutory requirements of the target entity needs to be undertaken. A thorough review of material information is essential to determining the suitability of the match with the other entity before entering into a formal relationship. The level of detail for due diligence depends on the size and resources (outside accountants, auditors, lawyers) available to conduct a thorough review.

Affiliation Agreement

The affiliation agreement is used when one nonprofit corporation ("X") acquires another nonprofit ("Y") with X becoming the sole member of Y. The affiliation agreement should provide corporation X the opportunity to elect the board members of corporation Y and thereby take control of Y. With an affiliation, both corporation X and corporation Y remain as legal entities and should not lose their tax-exempt statuses. In the interest of protecting both corporation X and corporation Y, a termination clause can be inserted into the affiliation agreement for a quick and clear exit should the corporations discover that the affiliation does not work as planned.

Management Agreement

The management agreement is used when one nonprofit corporation takes over the operations of another nonprofit corporation to manage the ongoing functions and specifically back-office operations of the other. Due to economies of scale it often benefits one corporation to have another corporation manage the back office systems and provide streamlined services. The management agreement can be used in coordination with an affiliation agreement or can be used on its own for management of operations.

Asset Purchase and Transfer Agreement

An asset purchase can be utilized to accomplish merging nonprofit Y corporation into nonprofit X corporation without X assuming the liabilities of Y. The asset purchase transfers Y's assets to X in exchange for payment by X for the purchase of Y's assets.

Sample Letter to the Attorney General

This example offers a sample letter that counsel or other representative of the involved parties can send to an attorney general's office requesting consideration and approval of the merger, affiliation, or other proposed partnership.

Office of the Attorney General Handbook for Charitable Organizations

This guide is provided by the Commonwealth of Pennsylvania to give nonprofit senior management basic information about matters that affect charitable nonprofit organizations. Topics include the rights, responsibilities, and duties of nonprofit board members and senior leadership.

Sample Memorandum of Agreement

The memorandum of agreement establishes an agreement between the relevant parties to cooperate on some form of affiliation, typically to be discussed and agreed upon later through a more formal, binding agreement toward the end of the affiliation process. Its purpose is to clarify the written understanding of the agreement between both parties.

MUTUAL CONFIDENTIALITY AGREEMENT

THIS MUTUAL CONFIDENTIALITY AGREEMENT ("Confidentiality Agreement") is made and entered into as of _____, 20xx, by and between X, a X nonprofit corporation with its principal office and place of business at X, and _____ with its principal office and place of business at _____ _____.

The parties to this Confidentiality Agreement have determined to establish terms governing the confidentiality of certain information that one party may disclose to the other in connection with the consideration of a possible affiliation or similar transaction between the parties (the "Transaction") and the parties' evaluation of such information and consideration of such Transaction.

NOW, THEREFORE, the parties, intending to be legally bound, agree as follows:

1. For the purposes of this Confidentiality Agreement, "Confidential Information" means all nonpublic information in whatever form transmitted, whether written, electronic, oral or otherwise, relating in any way to the Transaction or the evaluation of the Transaction, including without limitation, the knowledge that a party is considering such a Transaction and any discussions, negotiations, or other facts related to such Transaction which is disclosed by one party ("Disclosing Party") to the other party ("Receiving Party").

   Confidential Information shall not include any information provided by the Disclosing Party which (a) is independently developed by the Receiving Party or lawfully received free of restriction from another source having the right to so furnish such information; (b) is or becomes generally available to the public without breach of this Confidentiality Agreement by the Receiving Party; (c) is or becomes generally known in the industry or geographic location of the Disclosing Party; (d) at the time of disclosure to the Receiving Party was known to such party free of restriction; or (e) the Receiving Party is required to disclose pursuant to subpoena or other governmental mandatory process, provided that before making such disclosure the Receiving Party shall use reasonable efforts to furnish the Disclosing Party prior notice of such impending disclosure.

In consideration of, and as a condition precedent to, the disclosure of Confidential Information by the Disclosing Party to the Receiving Party, the Receiving Party agrees that all of the Confidential Information shall be treated as proprietary, secret and confidential whether or not designated as such.

2. The Receiving Party shall not use or disclose any Confidential Information it receives from the Disclosing Party to any person or entity for any purpose other than the evaluation of the Transaction. The Receiving Party shall restrict access to the Confidential Information to those of its representatives, agents, advisors and employees who reasonably require access to such Confidential Information for the Receiving Party to evaluate the Transaction.

    The Receiving Party shall use not less than the same degree of care (but no less than a reasonable degree of care) to avoid disclosure of such Confidential Information as the Receiving Party uses for its own confidential information of like importance. The Receiving Party shall use reasonable efforts to ensure that Confidential Information and all materials relating to the Disclosing Party at the premises of the Receiving Party or in the control of the Receiving Party shall be stored at locations and under such conditions as to prevent the unauthorized disclosure of such information and materials.

3. All Confidential Information disclosed by the Disclosing Party to the Receiving Party under this Confidentiality Agreement (including, without limitation, information incorporated in computer software or held in electronic storage media) shall be and remain property of the Disclosing Party. All Confidential Information in tangible form shall be returned to the Disclosing Party promptly upon termination of this Confidentiality Agreement pursuant to Section 12 and shall not thereafter be retained in any form by the Receiving Party. The rights and obligations of the parties under this Confidentiality Agreement shall survive any such return of Confidential Information.

4. The Disclosing Party shall not have any liability or responsibility for errors or omissions in, or any business decisions made by the

Receiving Party in reliance on, any Confidential Information disclosed under this Confidentiality Agreement. This provision shall not negate or limit any representations, warranties, or covenants.

5. The Receiving Party acknowledges that monetary damages may not be a sufficient remedy for unauthorized disclosure of Confidential Information and that the Disclosing Party shall be entitled, without waiving any other rights or remedies, to seek such injunction or equitable relief as may be deemed proper by a court of competent jurisdiction.

6. Neither party shall in any way or in any form disclose, publicize or advertise in any manner the discussions that give rise to this Confidentiality Agreement.

7. This Confidentiality Agreement shall not be construed to grant the Receiving Party any license or other rights to any information disclosed to it by the Disclosing Party.

8. Subject to the limitations set forth in this Confidentiality Agreement, this Confidentiality Agreement shall be binding upon and inure to the benefit of the parties and their respective affiliates, successors, and assigns.

9. This Confidentiality Agreement: (a) is the complete agreement between the parties concerning the parties' confidentiality obligations with respect to information disclosed to the other related to the Transaction and supersedes any prior such agreements with respect to information disclosed to the other related to the Transaction; (b) may not be amended or in any manner modified except in writing signed by the parties; and (c) shall be governed by and construed in accordance with the laws of the Commonwealth of Pennsylvania without regard to its choice of law provisions and the parties shall be subject to the exclusive jurisdiction of the state and federal courts located in the Commonwealth of Pennsylvania. If any provision of this Confidentiality Agreement is found to be unenforceable, the remainder shall be enforced as fully as possible and the unenforceable provision shall be deemed modified to the limited extent required to permit its enforcement in a manner most closely approximating the intention of the parties as expressed herein.

10. Each party expressly agrees that except as may be provided in a final definitive agreement regarding the Transaction or other agreement

executed by both parties, neither party shall have any obligation to enter into any transaction with the other party whether regarding affiliation or otherwise. Each party reserves the right, in its sole discretion, to reject any and all proposals made by the other party with regard to the Transaction and to terminate discussions and negotiations with the other party at any time.

11. Any notices, requests, demands, and other communications hereunder shall be deemed to have been duly given upon receipt and may be given by personal delivery, certified mail, or commercial overnight delivery service to the addresses listed above or such other address of which either party may notify the other.

12. This Confidentiality Agreement and any rights of the parties to obtain and retain Confidential Information provided pursuant to this Confidentiality Agreement may be terminated (i) by either party at any time upon written notice to the other party of such party's intention to terminate this Confidentiality Agreement or (ii) upon the execution of a definitive agreement regarding the Transaction. Notwithstanding the foregoing, this Agreement shall expire ninety (90) days from the date of execution. The parties may extend the term by a writing signed by both parties. The rights and obligations hereunder shall survive with respect to Confidential Information disclosed prior to termination for a period of one (1) year from the date of termination.

13. This Confidentiality Agreement may be executed and delivered by facsimile, or other electronic means, in counterparts, each of which when so executed shall be deemed to be an original and both of which when taken together shall constitute one agreement.

IN WITNESS WHEREOF, the parties have executed this Confidentiality Agreement as of the date first above written.

X Corporation   Y Corporation

By: _____   By: _____

Printed Name: _____   Printed Name: _____

Title: _____   Title: _____

AFFILIATION FEASIBILITY ASSESSMENT

Organization: _____

Executive Director: _____

Total Budget: $ _____

	Yes		Neutral		No
	1	2	3	4	5
Organization has had positive net revenue over the last 3 years					
Organization supports PHMC mission/vision					
PHMC has the capacity to address the needs of the organization					
Affiliation would expand our fundraising opportunities					
Organization's infrastructure is sufficiently in place					
Level of risk management is reasonable					
Geographic focus includes PA, southern NJ, and DE					
Organization enhances referral and growth possibilities for PHMC					
Organization leader/staff enhances growth possibilities for PHMC					

Affiliation Information to Request

- ✓ Program information
- ✓ The three most recent audits
- ✓ Recent financial statements
- ✓ Staffing and organizational charts, etc.
- ✓ Capital and equipment budgets
- ✓ Current operating budget
- ✓ Revenue streams and reimbursement rates
- ✓ Contracts and grants (contract summary)
- ✓ Loan and credit agreements from all bank lines, loans, debt instruments, guarantees with letter of credit, etc.
- ✓ Description of qualified and unqualified benefit, profit-sharing, and pension plans
- ✓ Any self-funded insurance coverage

DUE DILIGENCE REQUEST LIST

In connection with the potential acquisition of [NAME OF TARGET] (together with all of its subsidiaries, affiliates, and any predecessors, collectively, the "Nonprofit"), please provide us with the following materials. If certain materials have already been provided or are unavailable or inapplicable, please indicate so in your response to this request. Please note that our due diligence investigation is ongoing and that we will submit supplemental due diligence requests as necessary.

Unless otherwise indicated, documents should be made available for all periods subsequent to [DATE] and should include all amendments, supplements, and other ancillary documents. Unless otherwise indicated, the word "material" means an item involving payments (to or from the Nonprofit) or liabilities in excess or $[DOLLAR AMOUNT]. Please do not hesitate to contact us at [CONTACT INFORMATION] with any questions or concerns regarding this request.

1. Corporate Records.
   (a) Organizational documents of the Nonprofit and each of its subsidiaries and affiliates.
   (b) Books of the Nonprofit and each of its subsidiaries and affiliates, including minutes of meetings and actions by written consent of the board of directors (or its equivalent) of the Nonprofit and any of its committees.
   (c) Communications with members, including annual reports, statements, and correspondence.
   (d) Summary of the corporate history of the Nonprofit and any predecessors, including any mergers, acquisitions, changes in control, and divestitures.
   (e) Organizational structure chart of the Nonprofit and its subsidiaries identifying the legal name, type of entity, ownership, and jurisdiction of the organization.
   (f) List of current officers and directors, with resumes or biographies for each, including tenure with the Nonprofit.
   (g) List of all entities that are not subsidiaries of the Nonprofit but in which the Nonprofit owns an interest or has an affiliation.
   (h) List of places where the Nonprofit is qualified to carry out its purpose.

(i)   List of places where the Nonprofit operates or maintains, owns, or leases property or has employees, agents, or independent contractors. Include the number of employees and a description of operations or services performed at each location.

(j)   List and description of all transactions between the Nonprofit and any member, director, officer, employee, or affiliate of the Nonprofit (or any entity or person formerly having the status thereof), including amounts and names of parties involved, during the past [NUMBER] years.

(k)   Descriptions of any common interests and ownership between the Nonprofit, its officers or directors, and any supplier, vendor, or recipient of services.

2. Financing Documents.

(a)   Summary of currently outstanding short-term debt, long-term debt, inter-agency debt, contingent obligations, and capital lease obligations of the Nonprofit, including amounts, maturities, and prepayment terms.

(b)   Copies of any currently outstanding commitment letters or other correspondence relating to proposed financings or borrowings that may involve amounts in excess of $[DOLLAR AMOUNT] of indebtedness of the Nonprofit.

(c)   All correspondence and documents relating to contingent liabilities exceeding $[DOLLAR AMOUNT].

(d)   All documents purporting to create liens, mortgages, security agreements, pledges, charges, or other encumbrances on the stock of the Nonprofit, on any real or personal property of the Nonprofit or in favor of the Nonprofit. Copies of all Uniform Commercial Code financing statements filed with respect to the above.

(e)   Agreements evidencing borrowings by the Nonprofit, whether secured or unsecured, documented or undocumented, including loan and credit agreements, mortgages, deeds of trust, letters of credit, indentures, promissory notes, and other evidence of indebtedness, and any amendments, renewals, notices, or waivers.

(f)   Documents and agreements evidencing other material financing arrangements, including capital leases, synthetic leases, sale and leaseback arrangements, installment purchases, or similar agreements.

(g) All agreements pursuant to which the Nonprofit is or will be subject to any obligation to provide funds to or to make investments in any other person (in the form of a loan, capital contribution, or otherwise).

(h) Documents and agreements relating to any guarantees by the Nonprofit or releases of guarantees.

(i) Bank letters or agreements confirming lines of credit, including any amendments, renewal letters, notices, waivers, etc.

(j) Copies of notes payable to or notes receivable from any employee, director, affiliate, agent, or member of the Nonprofit outstanding at any time during the past year. Copies of all other financing agreements relating, directly or indirectly, to the Nonprofit or any person who is, or is proposed to become a member, officer, director, or key employee of the Nonprofit (including loans, leases, purchases, and sales of property).

3. Other Material Contracts.

(a) Any partnership, joint venture, distributorship, licensing, management, research and development, or similar agreements or contracts to which the Nonprofit is a party.

(b) Contracts with vendors and suppliers.

(c) List of the Nonprofit's suppliers (other than suppliers of goods and services generally required by all businesses, e.g. office supplies, utilities, etc., unless in excess of $[DOLLAR AMOUNT] from an individual supplier during any 12-month period) including for each supplier, indicating the amount and nature of products supplied.

(d) Material agreements relating to the sale or lease of the Nonprofit's personal property (including equipment) and any related financing arrangements.

(e) All material warranty and service agreements.

(f) Installment sales agreements.

(g) Any agreements between the Nonprofit and its affiliates or subsidiaries.

(h) Any material purchase agreements and other significant documents relating to any reorganization, any privatization transactions, mergers, or consolidations, in the past [NUM-BER] years or currently proposed.

(i) Any material purchase agreements and other significant documents relating to any acquisitions or dispositions by the Nonprofit in the past [NUMBER] years or currently proposed.

(j) Any indemnification agreements.

(k) Any other material agreements or drafts of proposed material agreements of the Nonprofit.

(l) Details of any material negotiations currently in progress.

4. Management/Employees.

(a) All corporate policy and employee manuals covering hiring, employee benefits, regulatory compliance, and internal controls.

(b) Organizational charts of management by department.

(c) Number of employees by department and by functional area.

(d) Copies of offer letters, employment contracts, bonus guarantees, severance agreements, change-of-control agreements, independent contractor agreements, nondisclosure and confidentiality agreements, noncompetition agreements, and management and consulting contracts.

(e) Any union contracts or collective bargaining agreements, and a summary of any ongoing negotiations with unions.

(f) Documents relating to all profit-sharing and savings plans, pension or retirement plans, supplemental retirement plans, retiree medical arrangements, deferred compensation plans, severance, medical, flexible spending, dental, or other health and welfare plans and any bonus, incentive, performance, or other employee compensation plans or arrangements, and related agreements (that provide benefits to current or former directors, officers, or employees and their respective beneficiaries); materials describing any of the foregoing or contemplated amendments, and the applicable trust accounting, IRS determination letter(s), Form 5500 filings, plan audit reports, actuarial reports, and other applicable financial statements for the three most recent years. Summary plan descriptions for each of the foregoing, to the extent available.

(g) Copies of all filings and correspondence with the IRS, the Department of Labor, and the Pension Benefit Guaranty Corporation (not covered in the preceding paragraph) made during the three most recently completed plan years.

(h) Copies of complaints and other material pleadings and court filings in connection with any pending lawsuit involving any employee benefit plan or benefits thereunder, or any such lawsuit filed within the past three years.

(i) Any notices or other communications issued within the past three years relating to blackout periods under any defined contribution plan or regarding any future reductions in medical, pension or other employee benefit or regarding the termination of any employee benefit arrangements.

(j) Cost/benefit information for each current plan for the most recent plan year, including (i) administrative costs, (ii) employer contributions, (iii) employee contributions, and (iv) benefit distributions.

(k) Copies of any Section 280G calculations performed with respect to potential parachute payments.

(l) Description of any threatened or pending labor disputes, work stoppages, work slowdowns, walkouts, lockouts, or union-organizing activities. Copies of any National Labor Review Board or U.S. Department of Labor filings.

(m) Any indemnification agreements with any directors, officers, employees, or agents.

(n) Schedule of all compensation paid during the last fiscal year to officers, directors, and key employees, showing separate salaries, bonuses, and noncash compensation, including bonuses paid or accrued, direct or indirect benefits or perquisites, and all benefits paid or accrued under all employee benefit plans.

(o) Description of commissions paid to managers, agents, or other employees of the Nonprofit.

(p) Copies of all agreements relating to arrangements securing in any way the payment of deferred compensation, severance, or other payments to employees or directors.

(q) A list of all outstanding loans to employees in excess of $[DOLLAR AMOUNT] (including loans granted under any

401(k) plan) including the amount of the loan, its rate of interest, and whether or not it is secured.

(r)   Absenteeism, disciplinary action, and accident records and turnover rates of the Nonprofit and its Subsidiaries.

(s)   Copies of any special compensation or retention arrangements in connection with the proposed transaction.

5.   Financial Information.

(a)   Historical financial statements for the last [NUMBER] years. Include summary of significant accounting policies used by the Nonprofit.

(b)   Interim financial statements prepared since the end of the most recent fiscal year.

(c)   Most recent projected financial statements (by month for current year and projections for next [NUMBER] years) including supporting assumptions.

(d)   Management letters or special reports by auditors and any responses.

(e)   Description of and reasons for any change in accounting methods or principles.

(f)   Copies of any compliance and internal control reports that may be part of, or in addition to, the financial statements.

(g)   Copies of the Nonprofit's investment policy.

(h)   Listing of accounts and donations receivable and identity of donors, including donors that have listed the Nonprofit as a beneficiary in their wills.

(i)   Descriptions of temporary and permanent restrictions on the use of funds.

(j)   Information on planned acquisitions, affiliations, and dispositions.

(k)   List of assets (fixed and unfixed).

(l)   Detailed explanation of any change in or disagreement with auditors on accounting and financial matters in the last [NUMBER] fiscal years.

6.   Real Property.

(a)   List of real property owned by the Nonprofit, including size, location, and use of each parcel. Provide documents of title,

title insurance, mortgages, deeds of trust, leases, and security agreements for these properties.

(b) Any appraisals or surveys of the Nonprofit's real property obtained within the past [NUMBER] years.

(c) Outstanding leases for real property to which the Nonprofit is either a lessor or lessee, including ground leases and sub-leases, estoppel certificates, and related subordination or non-disturbance agreements.

(d) Any option or development agreements involving real property to which the Nonprofit is a party.

(e) Certificates of occupancy relating to any real property owned or leased by the Nonprofit.

(f) List of all material encroachments, liens, easements, or other encumbrances on any real property owned or leased by the Nonprofit.

7. Intellectual Property.

(a) List of all U.S. and foreign patents and patent applications owned or held for use by the Nonprofit, indicating in each case, as applicable, the record owner, the dates of invention, application, issue, reexamination and reissue, the patent number or application serial number, and copies of all related prosecution files.

(b) List of all U.S. and foreign copyright (and mask work) regis-trations and applications owned or held for use by the Non-profit and material unregistered copyrights, indicating in each case, as applicable, the record owner, the dates of author-ship, publication, application, registration and renewal, the registration number, and copies of all related documents and files.

(c) List of all U.S. and foreign trademark, service mark, and trade name registrations and applications and all unregis-tered trademarks, service marks, and trade names owned or held for use by the Nonprofit, indicating in each case, as applicable, the record owner, the date of first use, appli-cation, registration and renewal, the registration num-ber or application serial number, and copies of all related prosecution files.

(d)   List of all domain names owned or held for use by the Non-profit, indicating in each case, the record owner, the registrar, and the registration and renewal dates.

(e)   List describing all proprietary technology and computer software owned, held for use by, or being developed by or for the Nonprofit.

(f)   List describing all:

    (i)   material third-party computer software used by the Nonprofit or incorporated into any software or product of the Nonprofit; and

    (ii) open source, freeware, or other software having similar licensing or distribution models to those used by the Nonprofit or incorporated into any software or product of the Nonprofit.

(g)   List describing all [material] trade secrets and other proprietary know-how or processes owned or held for use by the Nonprofit.

(h)   Copies of all [material] agreements, proposed agreements, or arrangements pursuant to which any third-party intellectual is assigned or licensed to the Nonprofit by any third party.

(i)   Copies of all [material] agreements and proposed agreements pursuant to which any intellectual property is assigned, sold, or otherwise transferred or licensed by the Nonprofit to any party or subject to a covenant not to sue.

(j)   Copies of all research and development, joint venture, or other agreements relating to product, process, or technical research, development, and testing to which the Nonprofit is a party.

(k)   Copies of all current and historical documents, policies, and procedures relating to the development and protection of the Nonprofit's intellectual property, including, without limitation, form invention and proprietary rights agreements.

(l)   Copies of all nondisclosure agreements, settlement agreements, administrative or judicial decisions or orders, consent orders, releases, covenants not to sue, security agreements, and other agreements or decisions restricting or encumbering the intellectual property of the Nonprofit.

(m) Copies of all freedom-of-use advice, validity, or infringement analyses and legal opinions of counsel regarding the intellectual property of the Nonprofit.

(n) Copies of all correspondence from third parties regarding alleged or potential infringement or other violation by the Nonprofit of the intellectual property rights of others.

(o) Descriptions of, and copies of all communications relating to, all:

   (i) pending or threatened claims, judicial or administrative proceedings, or litigation brought against the Nonprofit alleging the infringement or other violation of any third party's intellectual property or challenging the ownership, validity, or enforceability of the Nonprofit's intellectual property or any intellectual property exclusively licensed to the Nonprofit; or

   (ii) past disputes of such nature active in the last [NUMBER] years.

(p) Descriptions of, and copies of all communications relating to, all:

   (i) potential, pending, or threatened claims, judicial or administrative proceedings, or litigation brought or contemplated by the Nonprofit alleging the infringement or other violation of intellectual property of the Nonprofit or any intellectual property exclusively licensed to the Nonprofit by a third party or challenging the ownership, validity, or enforceability of a third party's intellectual property; or

   (ii) past disputes of such nature active in the last [NUMBER] years.

8. IT Systems and Networks.

  (a) Copies of all agreements relating to the provision of IT, data, or Internet-related products or services to or by the Nonprofit.

  (b) A description of all computer systems, software packages, networks and service bureaus ("Computer Systems") in use by the Nonprofit, by location.

  (c) Copies of the most recent strategic plans for the Nonprofit's Computer Systems.

(d) A description of any backup and disaster recovery arrangements, facilities management, and ongoing support arrangements, including details of service levels and charges.

(e) A description of and copies of documents relating to whether the Nonprofit has access, or rights of access, to the source code of material licensed software in order to ensure adequate maintenance and updating of said software.

(f) A description of any Nonprofit procedures to monitor compliance with the terms of software licenses, including whether said procedures monitor the use of software by the Nonprofit to ensure that multiple copies of any software are not used in breach of the relevant license terms.

(g) A description of and copies of the Nonprofit's website and Web services security policies and procedures.

(h) Confirm whether the Nonprofit owns all intellectual property in the design and content of its websites.

(i) A description of any insurance coverage for losses related to the Nonprofit's Computer Systems.

(j) A Description of any [material] interruptions of the Nonprofit's Computer Systems in the past [NUMBER] years.

9. Privacy and Data Security.

(a) Copies of all current and historical privacy and data security policies and practice manuals of the Nonprofit, including, without limitation, all privacy policies and procedures for the Nonprofit's use and disclosure of customer or personal information.

(b) Copies of all policies, procedures, and written information security programs for compliance with data protection and privacy legislation.

(c) Copies of all reports or audits (internal or external, including any SAS 70 and SSAE 16 audits) that have been performed on the Nonprofit's information security program(s) or any other reports prepared by or for the Nonprofit concerning the implementation of information security program(s).

(d) Copies of any other documentation and information regarding the Nonprofit's collection, use, storage, or disposal of customer or personal information (whether the Nonprofit's or a third party's).

(e) Copies of all agreements that the Nonprofit has with any third parties that act as the Nonprofit's agents or contractors and receive customer or personal information subject to any statutory or regulatory data privacy or security requirements from or on behalf of the Nonprofit. Please provide copies of any reports or audits (internal or external, and including any SAS 70 and SSAE 16 audits) that have been performed on the information security program(s) of said third parties.

(f) Details of any actual or potential data and information security breaches, unauthorized use or access of the Nonprofit's Computer Systems or data, or data and information security issues impacting the Nonprofit that have been identified in the past [NUMBER] years.

10. Environmental.

(a) Description of any Environmental Protection Act, Toxic Substances Control Act, or other investigation or claim.

(b) Environmental surveys, site assessments, or reports (including copies of any Phase I and Phase II reports) concerning any real property currently or formerly owned or leased by the Nonprofit.

(c) Environmental, health, and safety compliance verification reports (e.g., compliance audits) and quality assurance documents.

(d) Copies of any internal reports or memoranda prepared by the Nonprofit or third parties relating to hazardous materials, health and safety, or other environmental matters.

(e) Correspondence, memoranda, notes, or notices of violation from foreign, federal, state, or local environmental and health and safety authorities.

(f) Any "potentially responsible party" letters or other similar notices or requests for information from any governmental or regulatory authority.

11. Governmental Regulations and Filing.

(a) Summary of material inquiries by any foreign, federal, state, or local governmental agency.

(b) Copies of all contracts between the Nonprofit and any foreign or domestic governments (including regulatory bodies and other agencies with governmental authority).

(c) Status of foreign and domestic government contracts subject to renegotiation.

(d) Material foreign and domestic governmental permits, licenses, and certificates that the Nonprofit holds and their current status.

(e) List and description of all permits necessary for the Nonprofit to operate and carry out its purpose.

(f) Material filings made and significant correspondence by the Nonprofit with any state, federal, or foreign governmental or regulatory agencies since the Nonprofit's inception.

12. Litigation and Audits.

(a) List of all litigation for past [NUMBER] years.

(b) Letters from counsel sent to auditors for year-end for the past [NUMBER] years and current interim audits.

(c) Current list of all litigation, administrative or regulatory proceedings, investigations, or governmental actions involving the Nonprofit, with a brief description of the claim for each matter. Include name of court or agency in which the litigation proceeding is pending, date instituted, docket number, and principal parties to the action.

(d) Description of currently threatened litigation, legal claims, regulatory actions, or other actions or proceedings, including any correspondence relating to any threatened governmental investigation or alleged violation of law or regulation.

(e) Any currently effective consent decrees, judgments, other decrees or orders, settlement agreements, and other similar agreements to which the Nonprofit is a party or by which the Nonprofit or any of its assets is bound (or to which any officer or director of the Nonprofit is a party or by which any such officer or director or any of its assets is bound and which relates, directly or indirectly, to the Nonprofit).

(f) Correspondence, memoranda, or notes concerning inquiries from governmental tax authorities, occupational safety, health, and hazard officials, environmental officials, or authorities regarding equal opportunity violations, antitrust violations, or violations of any other law, rule, or regulation.

13. Insurance.
   (a) A schedule of all policies or binders of insurance or self-insurance arrangements, including medical, workers compensation, disability, automobile, general liability, fire and casualty, product liability, professional liability, business interruption, and officers and directors liability, with deductibles, coverage limits, and other significant terms. Please indicate the name and address of all insurance agents, brokers, and companies.
   (b) A schedule of insurance claims in excess of $[DOLLAR AMOUNT] over the last [NUMBER] years, and summary of loss history for such period.
   (c) Analysis of premium payments for the past [NUMBER] years and details regarding any cancellations or denials of insurance during this period.
   (d) Summary of self-insurance programs or other risk retention.
   (e) A schedule of threatened or potential claims.

14. *Taxes.*
   (a) Filed IRS Form 1023 (Application for Exemption) together with copies of all correspondence between IRS and the Nonprofit.
   (b) IRS determination letter.
   (c) Copies of Form 990, if any, and Form 990-T, if any, for the past [NUMBER] years.
   (d) Copies of any legal opinion(s) that may have been previously issued relating to the tax-exempt status of the nonprofit.
   (e) Copy of letter from IRS confirming that the Nonprofit is classified as a public charity, if applicable.
   (f) Copy of group exemption letter, if applicable.
   (g) Federal, state, local, and foreign tax returns for all open tax years, including sales, property, franchise, payroll, excise, withholding, and capital tax returns of the Nonprofit. Copies of tax elections, consents, agreements, or waivers (other than as attached to tax returns).
   (h) Information with respect to any foreign, IRS, state, or local tax examination or audit of the Nonprofit's or any of its

subsidiaries' or their respective affiliates and predecessor's returns and the results of each audit.

(i)   Copies of all documents relating to pending tax litigation or any appeals process or hearing.

(j)   Correspondence between the Nonprofit and the IRS or any foreign or state or local tax authority.

(k)   Description of any undertakings given by the Nonprofit to tax authorities or any special tax rulings or agreements arranged with tax authorities.

(l)   Any notices, elections, or other correspondence with foreign, federal, state, and local tax authorities regarding the reorganization of the Nonprofit and its predecessors to the extent material.

(m)   Copies of correspondence from outside tax advisors and accountants for the past three years.

AFFILIATION AGREEMENT

THIS AGREEMENT, made this day of, 20__, by and between _____ ("_____"), a Pennsylvania nonprofit corporation, and _____, a Pennsylvania nonprofit corporation.

Witnesseth

_____ is a nonprofit corporation engaged in the conduct and management of activities relating to health care and the delivery and improvement of health care services, and _____ is a nonprofit 501(c)(3) engaged in, among other things, _____. The parties desire to affiliate with each other, under and subject to terms and conditions of this Agreement, as a result of which _____ will become the sole member and parent of _____.

NOW, THEREFORE, the parties hereto, in consideration of the foregoing and of the mutual covenants contained herein, and intending to be legally bound hereby, agree as follows:

1. Affiliation. Subject to the terms of this Agreement, _____ and _____ shall affiliate with each other so that, effective _____, 201__ (the "Effective Date"), _____ shall become the sole member and parent of _____, and _____ shall become the membership subsidiary of _____.
2. Articles and Bylaws.
   A. Effective not later than the Effective Date, _____ shall cause its Articles of Incorporation ("the Articles") to be amended to provide that _____ shall be _____'s sole member by amending and restating the Articles in the form of *Exhibit A*.
   B. _____ shall cause its Bylaws to be amended so that the Bylaws attached to this Agreement as *Exhibit B* are the Bylaws ("the Bylaws") of _____ in effect on the Effective Date.
3. Management Agreement. _____ acknowledges that as of the Effective Date, _____ and _____ will enter into a mutually agreeable management agreement, pursuant to which _____ shall provide services to _____, as more fully described in the management agreement.

4. Board of Directors. Each current member of the Board of Directors of _____ shall sign a letter resigning effective as of the filing of the amendment to the Articles contemplated in Section 2(A). Thereafter, in its capacity as sole Member of _____, _____ will take appropriate action such that the representatives of _____ selected by _____, which may include current Directors of _____, pursuant to the Bylaws in effect on the Effective Date, shall constitute _____'s Board of Directors as of the Effective Date.

5. Credit for Service Time. _____ agrees that for all purposes (including vesting, eligibility to participate, severance, benefit accrual, and benefit level) under the employee benefit plans of _____ that provides benefits to any employee of _____, as of the Effective Date, each such employee shall be credited with his or her years of service with _____ before the Effective Date to the extent to which said employee was entitled, before the Effective Date, to credit for said service under any similar employee benefit plan of _____ in which said employee participated or was eligible to participate immediately prior to the Effective Date.

6. Use of Donor-Restricted Funds. _____ shall ensure that _____'s current donor-restricted funds will be used solely to support _____, in a manner that is consistent with any current restrictions on such funds.

7. Warranties. _____ represents and warrants to _____ as follows:

    A. _____ is a nonprofit corporation duly organized and validly existing and subsisting under the laws of the Commonwealth of Pennsylvania and has all requisite corporate power and authority to carry on its activities and to execute, deliver, and perform this Agreement and the transactions and affiliation contemplated hereby. This Agreement has been duly authorized by the proper corporate action of _____ and constitutes the valid and binding obligation of _____, enforceable against _____ in accordance with its terms.

    B. _____ is exempt from federal income taxes as a public charity under Sections 501(c)(3) and 509(a) of the Internal Revenue Code of 1986 and is duly registered as a charitable organization with the Pennsylvania Department of State Bureau of

Charitable Organizations. Such status is not currently subject to, and to the best of _____'s knowledge is not threatened to be made subject to, any administrative or other proceeding by the IRS or any other government agency.

8. Warranties. _____ represents and warrants to _____ as follows:

A.   _____ is a nonprofit corporation duly organized and validly existing and subsisting under the laws of the Commonwealth of Pennsylvania and has all requisite corporate power and authority to carry on its activities and to execute, deliver, and perform this Agreement and the transactions and the affiliation contemplated hereby. This Agreement has been duly authorized by all proper corporate action of _____ and constitutes the valid and binding obligation of _____, enforceable against _____ in accordance with its terms.

B.   _____ is exempt from federal income taxes as a public charity under Sections 501(c)(3) and 509(a) of the Internal Revenue Code of 1986, as amended, and is duly registered as a charitable organization with the Pennsylvania Department of State Bureau of Charitable Organizations. Such status is not currently subject to, and to the best of _____'s knowledge, is not threatened to be made subject to, any administrative or other proceeding by the Internal Revenue Service or any other government agency.

C.   _____ does not have, and since the date of its incorporation has never had, any members as defined in Section 5103 of the Pennsylvania Nonprofit Corporation Law of 1988, as amended, including specifically any members entitled to vote on any matter.

D.   The execution, delivery, and performance of this Agreement by _____ and the completion of the transactions contemplated by this Agreement do not and will not result in or constitute a conflict, violation, breach, or default (or an event that, with notice or lapse of time or both, would constitute a default), or give rise to any right of termination, cancellation, or acceleration under any of the terms, conditions, or provisions of any contract or other instrument or obligation to which _____ is a party or by which _____ may be bound.

9. No Assumption of Liabilities. The affiliation provided for in this Agreement extends only to the establishment of _____ as _____'s sole member, with each party retaining its corporate identity. Neither party is assuming or intends to assume any of the liabilities or obligations of the other party under any circumstances, and no such assumption of liability shall be implied.

10. Further Assurances and Cooperation. Each party shall take such action, execute and deliver such documents, and provide such cooperation as the other party may reasonably request to effectuate the terms of this Agreement and the transactions contemplated hereby, with the least reasonably practicable disruption to the business and affairs of the parties.

11. General Terms.

    A. The paragraph headings of this Agreement are for convenience of reference only and do not form a part of the terms and conditions of this Agreement or give full notice thereof.

    B. Neither party may assign or transfer all or any portion of this Agreement, voluntarily, involuntarily, by operation of law, or otherwise, without the prior written consent of the other party, and any attempted assignment or transfer to the contrary shall be null and void and have no effect.

12. Entire Agreement. This Agreement contains the entire understanding between the parties with respect to the subject matter hereof, and may not be amended or modified in any manner except by a written agreement duly executed by the party to be charged.

13. Notices. All notices, requests, consents, and other communications hereunder shall be in writing and shall be addressed to the receiving party's address set forth below or to such other address as a party may designate by notice hereunder, and shall be delivered (i) by hand, (ii) by a nationally recognized overnight courier, or (iii) by first class, registered, or certified mail, return receipt requested, postage prepaid.

If to _____:

If ____: _____

Attention: Executive Director

14. All notices, requests, consents, and other communications hereunder shall be deemed to have been given upon receipt, except that if sent by certified or registered mail, the date of delivery shall be the date of delivery specified on the receipt.

15. Governing Law. This Agreement shall be governed by and construed in accordance with the laws of the Commonwealth of Pennsylvania, without reference to principles of conflict of laws.

16. Severability. Any term or provision of this Agreement that is invalid or unenforceable shall be ineffective to the extent of such invalidity or unenforceability without rendering invalid or unenforceable the remaining terms and provisions of this Agreement. In all such cases, the parties shall use their commercially reasonable efforts to substitute a valid, legal, and enforceable provision that, insofar as practicable, implements the original purposes and intents of this Agreement.

17. No Third-Party Beneficiaries. This Agreement does not create, and shall not be construed as creating, any rights enforceable by any person not a party to this Agreement.

18. Counterparts; Delivery by Facsimile. This Agreement may be executed in counterparts and by each party hereto on a separate counterpart, both of which when so executed shall be deemed to be an original and both of which taken together shall constitute one and the same agreement. Delivery of an executed counterpart of a signature page to this Agreement by email or facsimile transmission shall be effective as delivery of a manually executed counterpart of this Agreement.

IN WITNESS WHEREOF, the parties have executed this Agreement as of the day and year first above written.

_____

                                              _____

By: _____   By: _____
Date: _____   Date: _____

BYLAWS

1. OFFICES
    (a)   Registered Office. The registered office of the corporation shall be at such place within the Commonwealth of Pennsylvania as the Board of Directors may from time to time determine.
    (b)   Other Offices. The corporation may also have offices at such other places as the Board of Directors may from time to time appoint or the activities of the corporation may require.

2. SEAL
    (a)   The corporate seal shall have inscribed thereon the name of the corporation, the year of its incorporation, and the words "Corporate Seal, Pennsylvania."

3. MEMBERS
    (a)   Sole Member. In accordance with the Articles of Incorporation, the _____ shall be the sole member of the corporation and is referred to in these Bylaws as the "Member."
    (b)   Annual and Special Meetings. The Member shall undertake annual meeting activity once during each calendar year. The Member may at any time undertake any other activity, such as would occur at a special meeting, by written consent.
    (c)   Notice, Quorum, Voting. To the extent procedural requirements regarding notice, quorum and voting apply, the Member shall proceed in accordance with applicable law.
    (d)   Designee. The Member may designate one or more individuals to act as the Member's designee for matters relating to the corporation. All the acts of such designee or designees shall be the acts of the Member for all purposes relating to the corporation, and the Board of Directors and all officers and representatives of the corporation shall be entitled to rely thereon.

4. BOARD OF DIRECTORS
    (a)   General Powers. The business and affairs of the corporation shall be managed by the Board of Directors, and all powers of the corporation not reserved to the member are hereby granted to and vested in the Board of Directors, except as

otherwise expressly provided in these Bylaws, the Articles of Incorporation, or by law.

(b) Composition, Selection, Removal and Vacancies.

    (i) There shall be not less than 5 and not more than 27 members of the Board of Directors, as the Member may determine after reasonable consultation with the Board, at least two of whom shall be representatives of the Member so designated by the Member.

    (ii) Members of the Board of Directors shall be selected by the Member. The Board of Directors may, by a nominating committee or such other procedure as the Board deems appropriate, make nominations or recommendations to the Member for the selection of directors to fill openings arising from the expiration of terms, increase in the size of the Board, vacancies in Board positions or otherwise. The Member shall review any such nominations and recommendations in good faith and act with due regard thereto; provided that, if the Board shall fail or refuse to act under this Subparagraph B in a timely manner, the Member shall select directors without the Board's nominations or recommendations and that all final decisions for the selection of directors shall be made by the Member in its discretion.

(c) Term. Directors shall serve for terms of not more than three years, as the Member may determine, and the Board may, with the concurrence of the Member, stagger terms so that one-half or one-third (or as close to one-half or one-third as possible) of the Board is elected each year.

(d) Regular Meetings. The Board shall hold at least three regular meetings each year at such times and places as the Board may determine by resolution.

(e) Special Meetings. Special meetings of the Board of Directors may be called, at any time, by the Member, the President or by one-third of the directors, by submitting a written request therefor, stating the object of the meeting, to the Secretary. The Secretary shall set the time and place of the meeting, which shall be held not later than 10 days after the receipt of the request. If the Secretary shall neglect or refuse to set the time and place of the meeting, the person or persons calling the meeting may do so. Business transacted at all special meetings shall be confined to the objects stated in the request therefor and matters directly related and germane thereto.

(f)   Annual Meeting. There shall be an annual meeting of the Board of Directors during the first calendar quarter of each year, or at such other time as the Board may determine. At the annual meeting, the directors shall elect officers, and transact such other business as may be properly brought before the meeting.

(g)   Notices. Written notice of regular and annual meetings of the Board of Directors, stating the time and place thereof, shall be given to all directors at least five days prior to the date of the meeting. Written notice of special meetings of the Board of Directors shall be given to each director at least 48 hours prior to the time of the meeting and shall state the business to be transacted at the meeting.

(h)   Quorum. One-third of the members of the Board of Directors shall constitute a quorum for the transaction of business. In the event that a quorum is not present at any meeting of the Board of Directors, the directors present may adjourn the meeting without any notice of the time and place of the adjourned meeting except for announcement at the meeting at which adjournment is taken.

(i)   Removal and Resignation.

The Member may remove any director at any time, with or without cause. If the Member proposes to remove a director pursuant to this Paragraph 4.9, it shall so notify the President and Secretary in writing. For a period of 14 days after the giving of such notice, the President or his or her designee or designees may discuss with the Member the proposed removal and make such recommendations to the Member concerning the removal as the President or designee deems appropriate. The Member shall provide the President or the designee with a reasonable opportunity to make recommendations, shall consider any such recommendations in good faith and shall make its decision and act on the proposed removal within a reasonable time after the expiration of the 14-day period provided for in this Subparagraph; provided that the decision with respect to the removal of a director shall be made by the Member in its sole discretion and shall be final and binding on all parties in all respects.

(i) The Board may at any time notify the Member in writing that the Board recommends that a director be removed from the Board, with or without cause. The Member shall provide the President or other designated representative of the Board with a reasonable opportunity to discuss the recommendation, shall consider the recommendation in good faith and shall act on the recommendation reasonably promptly after receiving notice thereof, provided that the Member shall determine in its sole discretion whether to remove the director in accordance with the recommendation, and the Member's decision shall be final and binding on all parties in all respects.

(ii) A director may resign at any time by submitting a written resignation to the President, or in the case of the resignation of a director who serves as President, to any other officer. A resignation need not be accepted to be effective.

(j) Compensation. Members of the Board shall not receive any salary for their services as directors, but directors may be reimbursed for expenses incurred in connection with service on the Board. Directors shall not be precluded from serving the corporation in any other capacity and receiving compensation therefor.

(k) Conflicts of Interest. The Board of Directors shall have the authority to establish, and from time to time amend, a policy concerning disclosing and dealing with actual, potential or apparent conflicts of the interests of directors with the interests of the corporation, which policy shall at all times conform to applicable law. The Board shall keep the Member advised of any action with respect to a conflict of interest policy, and any such policy shall be subject to revision by the Member.

5. COMMITTEES

(a) Establishment. The Board of Directors may establish one or more standing or special committees, including without limitation an executive committee. Except as otherwise provided in these Bylaws, the Articles of Incorporation, or applicable law, any committee may exercise such powers and functions as the Board of Directors may from time to time determine. If the Board establishes an Executive Committee, the two representatives of the Member designated under Paragraph 4.2A shall be members of that committee.

(b) Committee Members. Except as the Board may otherwise determine, the President shall appoint all committee members and committee chairpersons and may appoint alternates for any member or chairperson of any committee. All members of the executive committee, if any, shall be directors. All other committees shall have at least one director as a member.

6. OFFICERS

(a) Officers. The officers of the corporation shall be chosen by the Board of Directors and shall be a President, a Treasurer, a Secretary, and such Vice Presidents and assistant officers as the Board of Directors may determine that the needs of the corporation require. All officers shall be natural persons of full age and the President, Vice Presidents, if any, Treasurer, and Secretary shall be directors.

(b) Selection. The President, Treasurer and Secretary shall be elected by the Board of Directors at its annual meeting and shall serve for a term of one year. All Vice Presidents and assistant officers shall be elected or appointed at such times and for such terms as the Board of Directors may determine. Any vacancy in any office shall be filled by the Board.

(c) Authority and Duties. The President shall preside at all meetings of the Board of Directors. In all other respects, the officers shall have such authority and such duties and responsibilities as are customarily associated with their offices and performed and undertaken by officers of nonprofit corporations.

(d) Assistant Officers. Assistant officers shall perform such duties and have such responsibilities as the Board of Directors may from time to time determine.

7. LIMITATION OF LIABILITY AND INDEMNIFICATION

(a) Limitation of Liability. Directors of this corporation shall not be personally liable for monetary damages as such for any action other than as expressly provided in 15 Pa. C.S. §§513 and 5713. It is the intention of this Section 7.1 to limit the liability of directors of this corporation to the fullest extent permitted by 15 Pa. C.S. §§513 and 5713 or by any other present or future provision of Pennsylvania law.

(b) Indemnification. The corporation shall indemnify each director and officer, and may indemnify any employee or agent, to the full extent permitted by the Pennsylvania Nonprofit Corporation Law of 1988 and any other present or future provision of Pennsylvania law. The corporation shall pay and advance expenses to directors and officers for matters covered by indemnification to the full extent permitted by such law, and may similarly pay and advance expenses for employees and agents. This Section 7.2 shall not exclude any other indemnification or other rights to which any party may be entitled in any manner.

8. NOTICES

(a) Form of Notice. Whenever written notice is required or permitted, by these Bylaws or otherwise, to be given to any person or entity, it may be given either personally or by sending a copy thereof by first class mail, postage prepaid, or by telegraph, charges prepaid, or by overnight express delivery service, charges prepaid, to the address of the appropriate person or entity as it appears on the books of the corporation or by telecopier to the appropriate number. If the notice is sent by mail or telegraph or overnight express delivery, it shall be deemed to have been given when deposited in the United States Mail or with a telegraph office for transmission or delivered to the overnight express delivery service. If the notice is sent by telecopier, it shall be deemed to have been given when confirmation by the recipient is received by the sender.

(b) Waiver of Notice. Whenever a written notice is required, by these Bylaws or otherwise, a waiver of such notice in writing, signed by the person or persons or on behalf of the entity or entities entitled to receive the notice shall be deemed equivalent to the giving of such notice, whether the waiver is signed before or after the time required for such notice. Except as otherwise required by law, the waiver of notice need not state the business to be transacted at nor the purpose of the meeting, except that the waiver of notice of a special meeting of the Board of Directors shall specify the general nature of the business to be transacted at the meeting. Attendance at any meeting shall constitute waiver of notice of such meeting, except where a person attends a meeting for the express purpose of objecting, at the beginning of the meeting, to the transaction of business because the meeting was not called or convened upon proper notice.

9. MISCELLANEOUS PROVISIONS

(a) Fiscal Year. The fiscal year of the corporation shall be as the Board of Directors may determine.

(b) Participation by Telecommunications. One or more persons may participate in a meeting of the Board of Directors or of any committee by means of a conference telephone or similar communications equipment by which all persons participating in the meeting can hear one another. Participation in a meeting pursuant to this section shall constitute the presence in person at such meeting.

10. AMENDMENTS

(a) Amendments. Subject to the provisions of this Paragraph 10.1, the Member may amend or repeal all or any portion of these Bylaws at any time. If the Member proposes to take any action for the amendment or repeal of all or a portion of these Bylaws, it shall so notify the President and Secretary in writing, describing the proposed action. For a period of 14 days after the giving of such notice, the President, or his or her designee or designees, may discuss with the Member the proposed action and make such recommendations to the Member as the President or his or her designee deems appropriate.

The Member shall provide the President or the designee with a reasonable opportunity to make recommendations, shall consider any such recommendations in good faith and shall make its decision on the proposed action within a reasonable time after the 14-day period provided for in this Subparagraph; provided that the decision as to the proposed action to amend or repeal all or a portion of the Bylaws shall be made by the Member in its sole discretion and shall be final and binding on all parties in all respects.

(i)   The Board of Directors may at any time notify the Member in writing that the Board proposes to amend or repeal all or a portion of these Bylaws. The Member shall consider any such recommendations in good faith and provide an opportunity for the President, or another designee of the Board, to discuss the recommendation; provided that the Member shall determine in its sole discretion whether to take the recommended action, and the Member's decision shall be final and binding on all parties in all respects.

MANAGEMENT AGREEMENT

Between

_____

And

_____

THIS AGREEMENT, effective as of _____ by and between _____ (hereafter referred to as "_____"), a Pennsylvania nonprofit corporation, and _____ (hereafter referred to as "_____"), a Pennsylvania nonprofit corporation.

Witnesseth

_____ conducts certain programs and activities (collectively "the Programs") and is a wholly owned nonprofit membership corporation with _____ as its affiliate. _____ is engaged in providing assistance with health care activities and programs, and the parties desire to enter into this Agreement for _____ to provide technical and other assistance to _____ for the Programs, under and subject to the terms and conditions set forth herein.

NOW, THEREFORE, the parties hereto, in consideration of the foregoing and of the mutual covenants contained herein, and intending to be legally bound hereby, agree as follows:

1. Services. During the term of this Agreement, _____ shall perform the services relating to the Programs described on Attachment "A" hereto ("the Services").
2. Other Services. The parties may, at any time and from time to time, by a written agreement or instrument executed by both parties, provide for additional services to be performed by _____ for or relating to _____ or to add to or expand the scope of the Services provided for in Attachment A: Work Statement for such additional consideration and under such other terms as the

parties deem appropriate. Except as otherwise provided in the agreement or instrument signed by the parties, all such additional or expanded services shall be considered "Services" covered by and subject to all of the terms of this Agreement.

3. Exclusion of Executive and Management Authority. This Agreement and the activities of _____ hereunder are not intended and shall not be construed to relieve the Board of Directors, officers, or management of _____ of any authority, duties, or responsibilities.

4. Consideration. In consideration of the performance of the Services from _____ through _____, _____ shall pay to _____ a fee-for-service contract amount of $_____.

This amount is payable as follows:

1) For all Services and amounts, _____ shall submit to _____ monthly statements stating the fixed amount due for the month to which the statement applies. The statements shall be consistent with the FY14 management budget and in such form as _____ may reasonably determine. _____ shall pay the amount of each statement in full within fourteen (14) days after the statement is given;

5. Advance Funding of Operating Expenses and Costs. Due to _____'s status as a wholly owned nonprofit membership corporation with _____ as the sole member, _____ will at times fund in advance a variety of _____ 's ongoing operating expenses and costs. Such advance funding will be made at _____'s discretion and is limited to payments for approved eligible program and operating expenses as determined by various government and contract budgets and payment arrangements. This facility is further limited by _____'s ability to borrow or otherwise secure funds. _____ will submit to _____ a monthly statement-indicating amount of funds advanced and the purpose and nature of said advances. Also, _____ will directly apply as payments or pay-downs towards said advances all government and other funds received on behalf of _____. _____ will charge _____ a

finance charge consistent with _____'s current borrowing arrangement under its line of credit and will credit _____ based on the current bank earnings credit rate provided to _____.

6. Performance. _____ shall use reasonable efforts to perform the Services, with a view to assisting _____ in the proper and efficient conduct and operation of the Programs, provided that _____ does not in any manner guarantee or warrant any aspect of the conduct or course of or completion of any Programs. _____ acknowledges that _____ is not responsible for the success or failure of all or any portion of _____'s business.

7. Warranties

   a. _____ represents and warrants to _____ that: (1) it has complied and will comply in all respects with all grant requirements and all other requirements of any other government agency with respect to the operation of the Programs funded or governed by an agency; (2) it has obtained and will maintain in full force and effect all licenses, permits, and approvals required for the operation of its businesses and the conduct of the Programs; (3) it has conducted and will conduct the Programs in compliance with all applicable federal, state, and local laws, regulations, and ordinances, and (4) all financial statements and information delivered or provided by it to _____ will be true, correct, and complete; will be prepared in accordance with generally accepted accounting practices consistently applied; and will accurately present the results of operations and the financial position of _____ during the periods covered.

   b. _____ represents and warrants to _____ that all financial statements and information delivered or provided by _____ to _____ will be true, correct, and complete; will be prepared in accordance with generally accepted accounting practices consistently applied; and will accurately present the results of operations and financial position during the periods covered.

8. Insurance. Throughout the terms of this Agreement, _____ shall maintain in full force and effect general public liability and property insurance and other insurance, with reputable insurance companies and reasonable limits of liability and terms, consistent with prudent practices in the trade for activities in the nature of the Programs. _____ shall, upon _____'s reasonable request, cause _____ to be named a co-insured under said insurance policies and cause the policies to provide that they may not be canceled or terminated without at least ten (10) days advance written notice of cancellation or termination to _____. _____ shall maintain in full force and effect liability insurance of the type generally carried by organizations providing similar management services, with reputable insurance companies and reasonable limits of liability and terms, consistent with prudent practices in the trade for activities in the nature of the _____'s services.

9. Term. The term of this Agreement shall be from _____ to _____ but the parties may extend this Agreement for such a period and under such terms as they deem appropriate by a written agreement or instrument executed by both parties.

10. Termination.

   a. Either party may terminate this Management Agreement, effective thirty (30) working days after giving written notice of termination if the other party breaches any provision of this Management Agreement in any material respect and fails to rectify such breach within ten (10) days after written notice thereof. This Management Agreement shall terminate immediately upon termination of the Affiliation Agreement between _____ and _____ as of the date hereof, with such consequences as the Affiliation Agreement may provide.

   b. Upon termination of this Agreement for any reason, each party shall have and may exercise all remedies available to it under applicable law, with no remedy being exclusive and all remedies being cumulative.

11. Indemnification. _____ shall defend, indemnify, and hold harmless _____ from and against any and all claims,

demands, losses, costs, damages, suits, judgments, penalties, expenses, and liabilities of any kind and nature whatsoever, including reasonable attorneys' fees, incurred by _____ arising out of or in connection with any aspect of _____'s businesses and activities, including without limitations any aspects of the Programs, except to the extent actually caused by _____'s negligence or intentional misconduct. _____ shall defend, indemnify, and hold harmless _____ from and against any and all claims, demands, losses, costs, damages, suits, judgments, penalties, expenses, and liabilities of any kind and nature whatsoever, including reasonable attorneys' fees, incurred by _____ arising out of or in connection with any aspect of _____'s businesses and activities, except to the extent actually caused by _____'s negligence or intentional misconduct _____.

12. Outside Activities. _____ acknowledges that _____'s regular functions include management of and assistance with health care activities and can extend to management services for facilities similar to _____ and programs and projects similar to the Programs. _____ agrees that such activities and functions of _____ shall not constitute a violation of this Agreement or any obligations of _____ to _____, so long as _____ does not engage in any activities during the term of this Agreement that cause _____ to have an interest in direct conflict with the proper conduct and completion of the Programs and the performance of the Services under this Agreement.

13. Applicable Law. The Commonwealth of Pennsylvania shall govern the validity, construction, interpretation, and effect of this Agreement.

14. Further Assurances. Each party shall, upon the reasonable request of the other party, take such action and execute and deliver such documents as may reasonably be necessary or appropriate to effectuate the terms of this Agreement and the transactions and relationship contemplated hereby.

15. Assignments. Neither party shall assign or transfer all or any portion of this Agreement, whether voluntarily, involuntarily, by

operation of law, or otherwise, without the prior written consent of the other party, and any attempted assignment or transfer to the contrary shall be null and void and of no effect.

16. Headings. The paragraph headings of this Agreement are for convenience of reference and do not form a part of the terms and conditions of this Agreement or give full notice thereof.

17. Entire Agreement. This Agreement contains the entire understanding between the parties, no other covenants or representations having induced either party to execute this Agreement. This Agreement may not be amended or modified in any manner, except by a written agreement duly executed by the party to be charged.

18. Notices. All notices, statements, and other communications required or permitted under this Agreement shall be in writing and shall be sufficiently given only if personally delivered, mailed by registered, certified, or first class mail, transmitted by a reputable express courier service, or transmitted by fax and confirmed by first class mail within 24 hours to the party to receive notice at the following addresses, or at such other address as party may, by notice, be reached:

If to _____:

All notices shall be deemed as given when received, except that notice by first class mail shall be deemed as given on the second business day after the notice is mailed.

IN WITNESS THEREOF, the parties have executed this Agreement, under seal, the day and year first above written.

(SEAL) _____

Attest: _____   By: _____

                             _____

(SEAL) _____

Attest: _____   By: _____

                             _____

ATTACHMENT A

MANAGEMENT CONTRACT
FISCAL YEAR 20__
WORK STATEMENT

A more detailed management contract will be developed in partnership with _____.

In general, _____ will provide the following technical assistance and management support services, including, but not limited to:

Executive Management Support

- Corporate-wide strategy support for _____ senior management and leadership
- Government and community relations and strategic support

Fiscal Management Support

- Assistance with budget development, negotiations, and general support for _____'s leadership
- Assistance with development plans

Human Resources

- Human resources technical assistance and general support
- Training
- Human resources integration

Program Development and Fundraising

- Proposal development in response to requests for proposals and other funding opportunities
- Fundraising development strategies
- Assistance in fundraising

- Grant management and administration
- Program development and guidance

Quality Assurance

- Quality assurance and management support
- Training and corporate compliance assistance
- Quality assurance integration with _____
- Standards of care
- Privacy and confidentiality consultation

Marketing and Communications

- Broad-based marketing and communications support
- Messaging and branding support
- Planning and support of _____'s external and internal communications
- Design support

Administrative Services

- Information technology support and technical assistance
- Help desk support

ASSET PURCHASE AND TRANSFER AGREEMENT

This Asset Purchase and Transfer Agreement ("Agreement") is entered into as of ___, ____ by and between _____, a _____ nonprofit corporation with its principal place of business at _____ ("Seller"), and _____, a _____ nonprofit corporation with its principal place of business located at _____ ("Buyer").

RECITALS

Seller operates and maintains a nonprofit corporation that _____

Seller desires to sell to Buyer and Buyer desires to Purchase from Seller the assets as set forth in Section 1 herein, which assets are related to the program provided by Seller, on the terms and conditions set forth in this Agreement.

Buyer intends to continue the operations of Seller as part of one of its programs.

NOW THEREFORE, for and in consideration of the promises, representations, and covenants in this Agreement, and other good and valuable consideration, the receipt and adequacy of which are hereby acknowledged, and intending to be legally bound hereby, the parties agree as follows:

SECTION 1 ACQUIRED ASSETS

Subject to the terms and conditions of this Agreement, on the Closing Date (as hereinafter defined), and to the fullest extent permitted by law, Seller agrees to sell, transfer, convey, assign, and deliver to Buyer, and Buyer agrees to purchase and accept all rights, title, and interest in and to, the following assets of Seller (hereafter "Acquired Assets"):

(a) the equipment, supplies, inventory, records, and other assets of Seller used in connection with the provision of residential care at Buyer's premises, as listed on Schedule 1, hereof, and to the extent assignable by Seller, any and all existing warranties (express or implied), and all rights and claims assertable by (but not against) Seller relating to such assets;

(b) all rights and interests of Seller in the contracts, commitments, leases, and agreements listed on Schedule 2 hereto (hereafter "the Contracts"), to the extent that said rights and interests are assignable, and to the extent that said rights and interests are not assignable, Seller agrees to use its best efforts to cause said rights and interests to be transferred to Buyer as promptly as possible.

(c) the lease between Buyer and _____ shall be assigned to Buyer. The salient terms of the lease include that Buyer shall pay a rent of _____ ($__) per month from _____ until _____, 201_.

(d) all rights and interests of Seller in the licenses and permits listed in Schedule 3 hereof ("The Permits"), to the extent assignable, held by Seller and relating to the provision of any and all services provided by Seller and to the extent such licenses and permits are not assignable, Seller agrees to use its best efforts to cause said licenses and permits to be transferred to Buyer as promptly as possible.

(e) all cash, cash equivalents, or accounts receivable ("Cash").

SECTION 2 OBLIGATIONS AND ASSUMED LIABILITIES

(a) In connection with the conveyance of the Acquired Assets, Buyer agrees to assume as of the Closing Date, the future payment and performance of Seller's obligations accruing after the Closing Date under the contracts assigned to and assumed by Buyer (the "Assumed Liabilities").

(b) Apart from the Assumed Liabilities, Buyer and its affiliates shall not assume any obligations or liabilities of Seller, and Buyer and its affiliates shall not be liable for any claim(s) from unsecured defaults in the performance of any and all Contracts for periods prior to the Closing Date or unpaid amounts in respect of the Contracts that are due as of the Closing Date or that relate to services rendered or goods provided before the Closing Date.

(c) Buyer agrees that it will not use for the purpose of billing for any services performed at Seller's operation after the Closing Date, or for the purpose of operating the program under any permits or licenses issued to Seller and not transferred to Buyer, any group identification number, employer identification number, or other tax identification number issued to Seller.

SECTION 3 PURCHASE PRICE

(a) Buyer shall pay the sum of _____ good and valuable consideration to Seller on the Closing Date.

SECTION 4 EXCLUDED LIABILITIES

(a) Buyer will not assume and under no circumstances shall Buyer be obligated to pay or assume, and none of the assets of Buyer shall be or become liable for or subject to, (i) any claims of malpractice or general liability relating to or arising out of acts or omissions of Seller occurring prior to the Closing; or (ii) except for the Assumed Liabilities, any liability, indebtedness commitment, or obligation of Seller, whether known or unknown, fixed or contingent, recorded or unrecorded, currently existing or hereafter arising (collectively, the "Excluded Liabilities").

(b) Seller shall retain all risk of loss of any sort and from any cause with respect to the Acquired Assets until Closing.

SECTION 5 CLOSING

(a) Subject to the satisfaction or waiver by the appropriate party of all the conditions precedent to Closing specified herein, the consummation of the transactions contemplated by and described in this Agreement ("Closing") will take place on or before _____, local time, on _____ ("Closing Date"), at the offices of _____ or at such later time and date or place as the parties may mutually designate in writing. If the Closing takes place on or before _____ on _____, the effective time and date of the Closing shall be 12:01 a.m., _____, and all transfers and assumptions, assignments, and deliveries shall be deemed for all purposes to be consummated at that time and on that date notwithstanding the fact that Closing is held prior thereto.

b) At Closing, unless otherwise waived in writing by Buyer, Seller shall deliver the following to Buyer: (i) a Bill of Sale, fully executed by Seller, conveying to Buyer the assets listed in Schedule 1; and (ii) an Assignment and Assumption Agreement fully executed by Seller, conveying to Buyer Seller's interest in the Contracts on Schedule 2 and the Permits listed in Schedule 3.

c) At Closing, unless otherwise waived in writing by Seller, Buyer shall deliver to Seller the following: (i) an amount equal to the Purchase Price; and (ii) an Assignment and Assumption Agreement fully executed by Buyer reflecting the assumption of the obligations under the Contracts listed on Schedule 2, subject to the limitations on said assumptions of liabilities by Buyer described in Section 4 above.

d) At Closing, unless otherwise waived by Buyer, transfer of all Cash and accounts receivable from Seller to Buyer.

SECTION 6 REPRESENTATIONS OF SELLER

As of the date hereof, Seller represents to Buyer, the following, which it believes to be true and correct:

a) Organization and Standing: Seller is a nonprofit corporation duly organized and subsisting in good standing under the laws of the state of _____.

b) Tax-Exempt Status: Seller is a _____ nonprofit corporation determined by the IRS to be exempt from federal income taxation pursuant to section 501(a) of the Internal Revenue Code of 1986, as amended ("Code") and described in section 501 (c)(3) of the Code. Seller has conducted its operations in a manner consistent with its tax-exempt status, has committed no act or deed that would cause revocation of its tax-exempt status, and has not received any letter or other notice of action, formal or informal, suspending, revoking, or threatening its tax-exempt status.

c) Authority to Enter Transaction:

    (i) Seller has the full power and authority to execute and deliver this Agreement and to perform its obligations set forth in this Agreement. This Agreement constitutes the valid and legally binding obligation of Seller and is enforceable in accordance with its terms and conditions.

    (ii) The execution, delivery, and performance of this Agreement by Seller and the consummation of the transactions contemplated herein by Seller:

        (1) to the best of Seller's knowledge do not require any approval or consent of, or filing with, any government agency or authority bearing on the validity of the Agreement that is required by law or the regulations of any said agency or authority, other than Attorney General approval;

        (2) to the best of Seller's knowledge, will neither conflict with nor result in any breach or contravention of, or the creation of, any lien, change, or encumbrance on or against the Acquired Assets under any indenture, agreement, lease, instrument, or understanding to which it is a party or by which it is bound.

        (3) to the best of Seller's knowledge, will not violate any statute, rule, law, or regulation of any government authority to which it or the Assets may be subject, having a material adverse effect on Seller or the Acquired Assets.

d) Title to Acquired Assets: Seller has the legal capacity and authority to transfer to Buyer the Acquired Assets as set forth on Schedule 1.

e) Litigation: Except as set forth on Schedule 6(e), Seller has no knowledge of any existing, pending, or threatened dispute, claim, action, suit, proceeding, arbitration, hearing, or governmental investigation, either administrative or judicial, relating to its management or operation of its business.

f) Compliance with Laws: To the best of its knowledge, Seller has complied with and is not in default under, or in violation of, any law, ordinance, rule, regulation, or order applicable to its operations, business, or properties that could adversely affect the Acquired Assets or the operation of its business.

g) Disclosure: To the best of its knowledge and the belief of the person signing this Agreement on behalf of Seller, no representations made by Seller in this Agreement contain an untrue statement of material fact or fail to state any material fact.

h) Insurance: Schedule 6(g) accurately discloses the insurance policies (including policy numbers, terms, identities of insurers, amounts, and coverage) covering the professional and general liability of Seller and the professionals who have worked at Seller's business during the four (4) years immediately preceding the Closing Date. All such policies are in full force and effect on an occurrence basis, and Seller has given in a timely manner to its insurers all notices required to be given under its insurance policies with respect to all of the claims and actions covered by insurance, and no insurer has denied coverage of any such claims or actions.

i) No Claims or Restrictions: Seller is not aware of any claims, assessments, security interests, liens, restrictions, or encumbrances against any of the Acquired Assets or any claims, actions, proceedings, or investigations pending or threatened against Seller or anyone else relating to Seller.

j) Attorney General Notification: Seller will provide all relevant notices and information to the Office of the Attorney General of _____ ("OAG") as required by the Review Protocol developed by the OAG for Fundamental Change Transactions Affecting Health Care Nonprofits, in order to permit the OAG to decide whether to object to or withhold objection to the transactions contemplated by and described in this Agreement. Buyer agrees to cooperate with Seller in preparing or providing any notices of documentation required by this section.

SECTION 7 REPRESENTATIONS OF BUYER

As of the date hereof, Buyer represents to Seller the following, which it believes to be true and correct:

a) Organization and Standing: Buyer is a nonprofit corporation duly organized and subsisting in good standing under the laws of the state of _____.

b) Tax-Exempt Status: Buyer is a _____ nonprofit corporation determined by the IRS to be exempt from federal income taxation pursuant to section 501 (a) of the Internal Revenue Code of 1986, as amended ("Code") and described in section 501(c)(3) of the Code. Buyer, to the best of its knowledge has conducted its operations in a manner consistent with its tax-exempt status, has committed no act or deed that would cause revocation of its tax-exempt status, and has not received any letter or other notice of action, formal or informal, suspending, revoking, or threatening its tax-exempt status.

c) Authority to Enter Transaction: (i) Buyer has the full power and authority to execute and deliver this Agreement and to perform its obligations as set forth in this Agreement. This Agreement constitutes the valid and legally binding obligation of Buyer and is enforceable in accordance with its terms and conditions.

d) Disclosure: To the best of the knowledge and belief of the person signing this Agreement on behalf of Buyer, no representations made by Buyer in this Agreement contain an untrue statement of material fact or fail to state any material fact.

e) Charitable Purpose: The Acquired Assets will be used by Buyer solely for charitable purposes.

SECTION 8 CONDUCT OF THE PARTIES PENDING CLOSING

a) General: Each of the parties hereto will use its reasonable best efforts to take all action and to do all things necessary, proper, or advisable in order to consummate Buyer's acquisition of the Acquired Assets in accordance with this Agreement (the "Transaction") by the Closing Date.

b) Conduct of Business: During the period between the execution of this Agreement and the closing Date, Seller will carry on its business in the ordinary manner and refrain from any action that would result in the breach of this Agreement.

c) Notice of Developments: Each party hereto will give prompt written notice to the other parties of any material adverse development that would affect its ability to consummate its obligations in accordance with the Agreement or any new information or changes of status that would make said party unable to make the representations and warranties at Closing.

d) Access: During the period between the execution of this Agreement and the Closing Date, Buyer will have access at all reasonable times to review, inspect, and copy all of Seller's books, records, contracts, and documents, and the books, records, contracts, and documents prepared and/or maintained by Seller's employees and relating to its operations. Seller will furnish or cause to be furnished to Buyer all information regarding the Acquired Assets reasonably requested by Buyer. Prior to Closing, all such information shall be held confidential by Buyer. In the event that this Agreement is terminated without Closing, said information will remain confidential and will not be used by Buyer or its officers, directors, employees, or agents (except as may be required by law), and all copies of said information will be returned to Seller.

e) Contracts and Commitments: During the period between the execution of this Agreement and the Closing Date, Seller will not enter into any contract, commitment, or transaction relating to Seller without the prior written consent of Buyer, which consent shall not be unreasonably withheld.

f) Sale of Capital Assets: During the period between the execution of this Agreement and the Closing Date, Seller will not sell, convey, transfer, or otherwise dispose of any equipment listed on Schedule 1 hereof, other than in the ordinary course of business.

g) Liabilities: During the period between the execution of this Agreement and the Closing Date, Seller will not create any indebtedness or other fixed or contingent liability including, without limitation, liability as a guarantor or otherwise with respect to the obligations of others.

h) Insurance: During the period between the execution of this Agreement and the Closing Date, Seller will maintain all present insurance, if any, that covers its employees, any other persons working at its place of operations, and the Acquired Assets.

i) No Default: During the period between the execution of this Agreement and the Closing Date, Seller will not commit any act or fail to do any act, or permit any act or failure to act that will cause a material breach of any contract, commitment, or obligation by which it is bound.

j) Tail Insurance: If any of the persons working for Seller prior to Closing (collectively, "Seller's Personnel") were not covered for professional and/or general liability by an occurrence policy, Seller will obtain, prior to Closing, at its sole cost and expense, an extended reporting claims endorsement ("Tail Coverage") to ensure that Seller's Personnel are fully covered for claims arising from acts or omissions prior to Closing even if the claims are filed after the Closing Date.

SECTION 9 CONDITIONS PRECEDENT
TO THE OBLIGATION OF BUYER

Notwithstanding anything in this Agreement to the contrary, the obligations of Buyer to consummate the transactions contemplated by and described in this Agreement are subject to the fulfillment, on or prior to the Closing Date, of the following conditions precedent unless, but only to the extent that, they are waived in writing by Buyer at or prior to the Closing:

a) Representations: Seller shall deliver a certificate that the representations made by Seller in Section 6 above shall be true and correct in all material respects on the Closing Date.

b) Performance of Agreements: Seller shall have performed and complied with all agreements and conditions set forth in this Agreement prior to or at Closing.

c) Adverse Change: There shall not have been a material adverse change, occurrence, or casualty, financial or otherwise, with respect to the Acquired Assets, whether covered by insurance or not.

d) Closing deliveries: Seller shall have delivered to Buyer prior to or at the time of Closing, the documents, assets, monies, and other items listed in Section 5 herein the Acquired Assets described in Schedule 1 of this Agreement.

e) No Litigation: There shall not be any threatened or pending action, proceeding, or investigation by or before any federal, state, local, or foreign court, arbitrator, or government body or agency that shall seek to restrain, prohibit, or invalidate the Transaction or that, if adversely determined, would result in a breach of any representation, warranty, or covenant contained in this Agreement.

f) Necessary Approvals: (i) Buyer shall have a fully executed Assignment of Lease entered into with _____ permitting Buyer to occupy and provide services at the premises where Seller is located; (ii) Seller shall cooperate with and assist Buyer and its representatives and counsel in obtaining any government and other approvals as may be required to consummate the Transaction as listed on Schedule 3.

Buyer may waive any condition specified in this Section by delivering a written statement to that effect to Seller at or prior to Closing.

SECTION 10 CONDITIONS PRECEDENT TO THE OBLIGATIONS OF SELLER

Notwithstanding anything in this Agreement to the contrary, the obligations of Seller to consummate the transactions contemplated by and described in this Agreement are subject to the fulfillment, on or prior to the Closing Date, of the following conditions precedent unless, but only to the extent that, they are waived in writing by Seller at or prior to the Closing:

a) Representations: Buyer shall deliver a certificate that the representations made by Buyer in Section 7 above shall be true and correct in all material respects on the Closing date.

b) Performance of Agreements: Buyer shall have performed and complied with all agreements and conditions set forth in this Agreement prior to or at the Closing.

c) Closing Deliveries: Buyer shall have paid the Purchase Price to Seller and shall have delivered to Seller the Assignment and Assumption Agreement as provided in Section 5 of this Agreement.

d) No Litigation: There shall not be any threatened or pending action, proceeding, or investigation by or before any federal, state, local, or foreign court, arbitrator, or government body or agency that shall seek to restrain, prohibit, or invalidate the Transaction or that, if adversely determined, would result in a breach of any representation, warranty, or covenant contained in this Agreement.

e) Licenses: Buyer shall have successfully transferred or obtained new licenses and permits as listed on Schedule 3 attached hereto, in its own name, in order to operate the program of Seller as of the Closing Date.

SECTION 11 MUTUAL OBLIGATIONS

a) Post Closing Access to Information: Seller and Buyer acknowledge that subsequent to Closing, one of the parties to this Agreement may need access to information or documents in the control or possession of the other party for purposes of concluding the transactions herein contemplated, audits, compliance with government requirements and regulations, the prosecution or defense of third-party claims, or other reasonable business purposes. Accordingly, the parties agree that for a period of six (6) years after the Closing Date, each will make reasonably available to the other's agents, independent auditors, and/or counsel and/or any government agencies upon written request and at the expense of the requesting party documents and information relating to the Acquired Assets for periods prior and subsequent to the Closing Date to the extent necessary to facilitate concluding the transactions herein contemplated, any audits, compliance with government requirements and regulations, and the prosecution or defense of third-party claims or other reasonable business purpose. Neither party has authority to make any statement, representation, or admission on the other party's behalf.

b) Preservation and Access to Records After the Closing: After the Closing, Buyer shall, in the ordinary course of business, and as required by law and the terms of this agreement, keep all records of Seller that constitute a part of the Acquired Assets delivered by Seller at the Closing. For purposes of this Agreement, the term "records" includes all documents, electronic data, and other compilations of information in any form. Buyer agrees to keep the client records delivered to Buyer at the Closing in accordance with applicable laws and regulations, and the requirements of relevant insurance carriers, all in a manner consistent with the maintenance of client records generated by Buyer after Closing. Upon reasonable notice, during regular business hours, at the sole cost and expense of Seller and subject to any restrictions imposed by law or regulation upon the Buyer, Buyer will afford to the representatives of Seller, including its counsel and accountants, full access to, and the right to make, at its own expense, copies of the records transferred to Buyer at the Closing (including, without limitation, access to client records relating to services provided by the program to clients prior to Closing). In addition, subject to any restrictions imposed by law or regulation upon Buyer, Seller shall be entitled, at its sole risk, to remove from the program copies made by Seller of any such client records, but only for purposes of a pending or threatened litigation or proceeding or government investigation or audit involving a client to whom said records refer, as certified in writing prior to removal by counsel retained by Seller in connection with said matter. Any access to the program or its records granted to Seller in this Agreement shall be on the condition that any such access not materially interfere with the business operations of Buyer and not violate any legal obligation imposed upon Buyer by law or regulation to limit or bar such access.

c) Employees: As of the Closing Date, Seller will have arranged with Buyer to transfer all employees of Seller listed on Schedule

11(c), and Buyer shall offer to employ all of said persons as employees of Buyer. After said transfer as of the Closing Date, the employment of said persons with Seller shall be immediately terminated by Seller. Buyer shall offer employment to said persons on substantially the same terms and conditions as they have been employed by Seller, and Seller shall deliver to Buyer at Closing a copy of the personnel records of all employees listed on Schedule 11(c), if such disclosure is authorized in writing by the employee who is the subject of the records. If said consent is not forthcoming by Closing, but is given after closing, Seller will deliver to Buyer the applicable personnel records within five (5) days after consent is received by Seller. Buyer will make reasonable best efforts to retain all salaries and benefits for the employees equal to or exceeding their previous salaries and benefits as of the Closing Date, including employee contributions to health care benefit plans. Employee leave balances and seniority for purposes of vacation and sick time shall transfer with the employee and be recognized by Buyer so that employees will not lose any vacation or sick time.

d) Misdirected Payments, etc.: Seller and Buyer covenant and agree to remit, within ten (10) business days, to the other party any payments received with respect to accounts or notes receivable owned by (or are otherwise payable to) the other. In addition, and without limitation, in the event of a determination by any government or third-party payer that payments to Seller resulted in an overpayment or other determination that funds previously paid by any program or plan to Seller must be repaid, or resulted in an underpayment that is due to Seller, Seller shall be responsible to pay said amounts (including defense of such actions) or receive said amount if said overpayment or underpayment determination was for services rendered before the Closing Date; Buyer shall pay or receive such monies (including defense of such actions) if such overpayment or underpayment determination was for services rendered after the Closing Date. Seller and Buyer each agree to remit, with reasonable promptness, to the other any charitable donations received that are intended for the other party. Upon the written request of the other from time to time, but no more frequently than once each calendar year, Seller and Buyer agree (1) to promptly provide to the other a list of all donations received during the prior twenty-four (24) months that are earmarked in whole or in part for the program, and (2) promptly to provide access to such information as may be needed by the other party to ascertain the contributor's intent in making each said donation. The list of donations shall include, among other things, the name of the donor, the amount of the donation, and the purpose of the donation.

e) Cooperation on Claims: The parties agree to work with each other to assist Seller to obtain information for payment of any outstanding claims to Seller post Closing.

SECTION 12 FEES AND EXPENSES

a) Expenses of the Transaction: The parties to this Agreement will pay their own expenses incidental to the preparation of this Agreement and the consummation of the transactions contemplated by and described in this Agreement.

b) Taxes and Expenses: Seller shall pay any sales, transfer, or documentary taxes or stamps, if any, that may be due as a result of the consummation of the Transaction.

SECTION 13 INDEMNIFICATION

a) Mutual Indemnification: Seller shall defend, indemnify, and hold harmless Buyer from and against any and all claims, demands, losses, costs, damages, suits, judgments, penalties, expenses, and liabilities of any kind and nature whatsoever, including reasonable attorneys' fees, incurred by Buyer arising out of or in connection with any act or omission of Seller's agents, contractors, or servants arising from this Agreement to the extent actually caused by their negligence or intentional misconduct. Buyer shall defend, indemnify, and hold harmless Seller from and against any and all claims, demands, losses, costs, damages, suits, judgments, penalties, expenses, and liabilities of any kind and nature whatsoever, including reasonable attorney's fees, incurred by Seller arising out of or in connection with any act or omission of the Buyer's agents, contractors, or servants arising from this Agreement to the extent actually caused by their negligence or intentional misconduct.

SECTION 14 TERMINATION

a) Termination of Agreement: The parties may terminate this Agreement as follows: (i) by mutual written consent at any time prior to the Closing Date; (ii) Buyer may terminate this Agreement prior to the Closing Date, if as a result of information discovered in its due diligence investigation, it determines in its sole discretion that completion of the transactions contemplated herein would be detrimental to its operations in any respect; (iii) Buyer may terminate this Agreement by giving written notice to Seller at any time prior to the Closing Date in the event Seller breaches any representation, warranty, or covenant contained in this Agreement, and Buyer has notified Seller of said breach and said breach has continued without cure for a period of five (5) days after the notice of said breach, or if any of Seller's representations or covenants are untrue, either as of the date of this agreement or as of the Closing Date. Seller may terminate this Agreement by giving written notice to Buyer at any time prior to the Closing Date in the event Buyer has (i) breached any material misrepresentation, warranty or covenant contained in this Agreement, and Seller has notified Buyer of said breach, and said breach has continued without cure for a period of five (5) days after the notice of said breach, or (ii) any representations or covenants made by the Buyer are untrue, either as of the date of this Agreement or as of the Closing Date.

b) Effect of Termination: Termination of this Agreement will halt and preclude any action to effect the transition of the program or the Acquired Assets to the Buyer, and will nullify any prior actions taken up to the date of termination.

SECTION 15 MISCELLANEOUS MATTERS

a) Arbitration: If any dispute arises under or in connection with this Agreement, it will be decided by three (3) arbitrators in an arbitration proceeding conforming to the rules of the American Arbitration Association applicable to commercial arbitration. The arbitrators will be appointed as follows: one by Seller, one by Buyer, and the third by the said two arbitrators, or, if they cannot agree, then the third arbitrator will be appointed by the American Arbitration Association. The third arbitrator will chair the panel. The arbitration will take place in _____. The decision by a majority of the arbitrators will be conclusively binding upon the parties, final and non-appealable except as provided by law, and said decision will be enforceable as a judgment in any court of competent jurisdiction. Each party will pay the fees and expenses of the arbitrator appointed by it, its counsel, and its witnesses. The parties will share equally the fees and expenses of the neutral arbitrator.

b) Governing Law: This Agreement is governed by and shall be construed and enforced in accordance with the laws of the _____.

c) Assignment: This Agreement shall not be assignable by either party without the prior written consent of the other party, except that Buyer may assign its rights and obligations under this Agreement without Seller's consent, to any of Buyer's affiliates or subsidiaries who agree to assume the obligations to Seller under this Agreement.

d) Headings: The section headings are for convenience only and shall not be interpreted to modify or limit the provisions of this Agreement.

e) Notices: Any notice or communication required or permitted to be given will be given by personal delivery, by registered or certified mail, postage prepaid and with return receipt requested, or by overnight mail by a nationally recognized overnight courier. Notice given by personal delivery will be effective upon delivery, and notice given by registered or certified mail or overnight mail shall be effective upon deposit. For notice purposes, the addresses of the parties are:

If to Seller:

If to Buyer:

With a copy to:

f) Schedules: The schedules to this Agreement are specifically made a part of this Agreement, and the representations made in such Schedules are intended to be binding on the parties.

g) Counterparts: This Agreement may be executed in any number of counterparts, each of which shall be deemed to be an original but all of which together shall constitute one and the same instrument.

h) Survival: The provisions of Sections 6, 7, 8, and 11 shall survive Closing.

i) Entire Agreement and Amendment: This agreement represents the entire Agreement of the parties with respect to the Transaction, and it supersedes all prior or contemporaneous Agreements, understandings, representations, and warranties between the parties. This Agreement may not be amended except by written instrument executed by the duly authorized officers of the parties.

l) Successors and Assigns: This Agreement shall be binding upon and inure to the benefit of the parties hereto and their respective successor and permitted assigns.

IN WITNESS WHEREOF, the parties have caused this Agreement to be executed and delivered on the day and year first written.

_____

Name

_____   _____

Title   Attest

_____

Name

_____   _____

Title   Attest

SAMPLE LETTER TO THE ATTORNEY GENERAL

Date _____

NAME
Senior Deputy Attorney General
Charitable Trust Section
Office of the Attorney General
21 South 12ᵗʰ Street, Third Floor
Philadelphia, PA 19107

RE: _____ Affiliation with _____

Dear NAME

I represent _____ ("_____"). The purpose of this letter and the attached package of information is to inform you of a proposed affiliation between _____ and _____ ("_____") and to request a determination that the Attorney General has no objection to the proposed affiliation.

_____ is a Pennsylvania nonprofit corporation that is exempt from federal income taxation as an organization described in section 501(c)(3) of the Internal Revenue Code (the "Code"). _____'s charitable mission is _____.

_____ is a nonprofit corporation that is exempt from federal income taxation as an organization described in section 501(c)(3) of the Internal Revenue Code (the "Code"). _____'s charitable mission is _____.

Both _____ and _____ have charitable missions directed at providing services to disadvantaged persons, and each desires to expand the services they are capable of providing. Through an affiliation, both parties will be able to leverage resources and collaborate more efficiently, thereby offering better service than either would be able to achieve alone. The affiliation will also enable both parties to be more responsive and better positioned to pursue opportunities in the _____region to help support people in need.

As a result, both organizations have engaged in negotiations over the past months, and each organization's board of directors has determined it advisable and in the best interest of each organization for the parties to formally affiliate, with _____ becoming the sole member of _____.

The terms of the proposed transaction are detailed in the agreement that both organizations signed on _____ (the "Affiliation Agreement"). The Affiliation Agreement is attached hereto as Appendix 1.

Accordingly, and pursuant to the Affiliation Agreement, upon receipt of a determination that the Attorney General has no objection to the affiliation, _____ will become the sole corporate member of _____. In anticipation of the affiliation and in an effort to operate more efficiently, the parties have entered into a management agreement attached hereto as Appendix 2. The management agreement details the back-office and support services _____ will provide to _____ for day-to-day operational matters, including in connection with the affiliation.

Extensive material is included for your review. A list of the materials contained in the accompanying binder is attached to this letter. The parties have negotiated in good faith, and their respective staffs have very good working relationships and look forward to an amicable transition as soon as possible.

After you have had an opportunity to assign this to your staff, I am available, as is _____, to answer any questions or clarify any information about the proposed transaction. Please do not hesitate to contact us if you need any additional information, or if we can help in any way to expedite the review by your office.

Respectfully
submitted,

OFFICE OF THE ATTORNEY GENERAL HANDBOOK
FOR CHARITABLE ORGANIZATIONS

Nonprofit Board Members and Senior Management:

The Office of the Attorney General recognizes the vital service that
you provide to your community through your work as a board
member or senior manager of a charitable nonprofit organization.
Your willingness to volunteer your time and expertise is deeply
appreciated.

The purpose of this guide is to provide you with some basic information about matters that affect charitable nonprofit organizations because those entities fall within the Attorney General's
jurisdiction. The Attorney General has a duty to protect the
public's interest in the charitable assets held by nonprofit
corporations.

In response to the many difficult questions confronting the boards
of charitable organizations today, the Attorney General's office is
offering this guide to assist you in your efforts to better serve your
organizations. This guide presents general information and is not
intended to direct the exact manner in which a Pennsylvania nonprofit board must operate.

To obtain additional information regarding your fiduciary duties as
a manager or board member or the rules and regulations for the
creation, operation and dissolution of nonprofit charitable organizations please consult the Nonprofit Corporation Law of 1988, as
amended, 15 Pa. C.S.A. §§ 5101–6162. This guide is not a substitute
for legal advice. If you have questions, seek qualified legal counsel
to ensure that you and your board's actions are in compliance with
Pennsylvania law.

Thank you for your hard work and dedication to public service. Our
Commonwealth is a better place because of your volunteer efforts.

INTRODUCTION

*This guide is intended to provide senior management and board members
with general information relating to the operation of charitable nonprofit*

organizations. If you have any questions regarding these organizations, please contact the Office of Attorney General at:

Commonwealth of Pennsylvania
Office of the Attorney General
Charitable Trusts and Organizations Section
14th Floor, Strawberry Square
Harrisburg, Pennsylvania 17120
Telephone: (717) 783–2853
Facsimile: (717) 787–1190
www.attorneygeneral.gov

QUESTIONS YOU SHOULD ASK BEFORE JOINING A BOARD

What is the charitable purpose of the organization?

Charitable purpose is defined by the Nonprofit Law as "[t]he relief of poverty, the advancement of education, the advancement of religion, the promotion of health, governmental or municipal purposes, and other purposes the accomplishment of which is beneficial to the community." Nonprofit Corporation Law of 1988, *as amended*, 15 Pa. C.S.A. §§ 5101–6162 (Nonprofit Law). Obtain as much information as possible about the organization. Review the Articles of Incorporation, bylaws, internal operating manuals, minutes of prior board meetings and annual reports.

What is the financial status of the organization?

As a board member or senior manager, you are responsible for ensuring that the assets committed to a charitable purpose are used for the charitable purpose for which they were intended. Review the nonprofit organization's financial statements and tax returns. Talk with the executive director, staff, and current board members if you have any questions about the finances of the organization.

What are my responsibilities as a board member?

Meet with the officers and executive staff of the charity to discuss your expected duties and responsibilities as a board member. Determine how much time you will be asked to commit to these duties. Ask about board committees, organizational structure, financial responsibility and conflict of interest policies.

OFFICERS AND DIRECTORS

Every nonprofit corporation must have a president, a secretary, and a treasurer. Although it is not necessary to use the above titles, every nonprofit corporation must have an individual who fulfills each of these roles and the same individual may fill multiple roles. In order to avoid the appearance of impropriety, it is best not to give one individual too much control over the corporation. Instead, power should be distributed among different officers or board members. A corporation may have as many officers with as many different titles as it deems necessary.

The bylaws may set forth the qualifications for the positions and the manner in which officers and directors will be elected. The length of the term that each officer or director will serve should be set forth in the bylaws. In the absence of a bylaw dictating term length, the Nonprofit Law provides that each officer or director will serve a one-year term. Committees may be established to handle some aspects of the organization's governance. At any time, an officer or director may resign by giving written notice to the corporation.

FIDUCIARY RESPONSIBILITIES OF BOARD MEMBERS AND SENIOR MANAGEMENT

1. DUTY OF CARE

Board Members, senior management, and members of committees must perform their duties in a manner they reasonably believe to be in the best interests of the corporation using the same degree of care, skill, caution, and diligence that a person of ordinary prudence would use under similar circumstances. Decision makers are required to make reasonable inquiries when analyzing contracts, investments, business dealings, and other matters. An individual who is acting in conformance with this standard will:

- attend and participate in board meetings on a regular basis;
- attend and participate in committee meetings when the individual is a member of the committee;
- diligently read, review, and inquire about material that affects the corporation;
- keep abreast of the affairs and finances of the corporation; and
- use independent judgment when analyzing matters that affect the corporation.

Decision makers may rely on information provided by their employees, committees, attorneys, public accountants, and qualified professionals as long as the decision maker reasonably believes that the information provided is reliable. Decision makers must use their own independent judgment when evaluating information. Individuals who fail to meet the prescribed standard may be personally liable to the corporation if their actions cause financial harm.

Board members, trustees, and senior management have a fiduciary responsibility when handling finances and investments. That simply means, they must exercise the degree of care, caution, and diligence that prudent persons would exercise in handling their own personal investments and finances. Individuals who have or claim to have special knowledge or skills in the area of investment will be held to a higher standard. Fiduciaries who carelessly or negligently invest funds may be personally liable for any losses sustained.

2. DUTY OF LOYALTY

Board members and senior management must always perform their duties in good faith with the best interests of the organization in mind. This means that they must not seek to derive private gain from business transactions that involve the nonprofit corporation or advance their own interests at the expense of the corporation. Acts of self-dealing constitute a breach of fiduciary duty which may result in personal liability to the nonprofit organization. Board members, trustees, and senior management should avoid conflicts of interest and even the appearance of impropriety. Individuals who take advantage of corporate opportunities to make profits for themselves at the expense of the corporation may be liable for the profits they received at the organization's expense.

CONFLICT OF INTEREST

Board members and senior management have a duty to avoid potential or apparent conflicts of interest. To avoid the appearance of impropriety, it is important for individuals to be open and honest with their fellow managers and board members at all times. It is particularly important for board members to disclose the following facts:

- whether they have a potential conflict of interest with respect to any transaction, business decision, or other matter in which the organization is involved;
- whether they have a financial, business, or personal interest in an entity with which the nonprofit organization is or will be doing business;
- whether individuals related to them have a financial, business, or personal interest in an entity with which the nonprofit organization is or will be doing business; or
- whether they serve as a director, member, or employee of either a competitor of the corporation or a corporation with which the nonprofit organization is or will be doing business.

The board should proceed with caution when any of the above facts are present because there may be a conflict of interest. An individual who has a potential conflict with respect to a particular transaction should disclose it to fellow managers and board members and abstain from participating in the negotiations and decisions surrounding that transaction. To avoid the appearance of impropriety, the individual who has the conflict of interest should not be present in the room during any discussions that relate to the transaction.

COMPENSATION FOR BOARD MEMBERS AND SENIOR MANAGEMENT

Board members and senior managers of nonprofit organizations are not always paid for their services and the bylaws should state whether any individual will be compensated. Individuals are not entitled to compensation unless a clear compensation agreement has been reached. The determination of whether or not to compensate individuals for their services is generally made by the board unless the bylaws provide otherwise.

In the event that compensation is received, the amount must be reasonable based upon the value of the services rendered; it must not be excessive. Compensation includes all salaries, commissions, bonuses, pensions, benefits, gifts, living expenses and all other perquisites and items of value of any kind. The level of compensation that is to be paid to each individual should be determined independently by the board of directors or a committee vested with the authority to set compensation. Individual employees should not be involved in setting their own compensation. In determining whether compensation is reasonable, the salary ranges of similarly situated individuals in similar nonprofit organizations should be examined.

A nonprofit organization may not compensate individuals who are not providing services to the organization. An organization's status as a nonprofit entity may be threatened if its employees receive excessive compensation or if individuals receive compensation without rendering services.

RIGHTS OF BOARD MEMBERS

- Board members have the right to receive all information that is necessary and relevant to assist them in performing their duties.
- Board members have the right to call special meetings by submitting written requests and once requested, a meeting must be held within the 60 days following the organization's receipt of the written request.
- Board members may bring court actions to contest activities that affect their rights and duties.

- Board members have the right to disagree with actions taken at meetings and may ask to have their disagreement noted in the minutes of the meeting at which the action was taken. Otherwise, they may submit a written dissent to the secretary of the corporation immediately following the meeting. However, board members may not dissent if they voted in favor of the action that was taken. It is important to note that board members who fail to note their dissent either in writing or in the minutes will be assumed to have assented to the board's action.

RIGHTS OF GENERAL MEMBERS

- The rights of general members of the nonprofit organization are governed by the organization's bylaws and the extent of the members' interest in the organization. For example, members who are entitled to cast at least 10% of the total membership votes are entitled to call special meetings by means of a written request. Once the written request is received, the meeting must be held within 60 days.
- Unless the members of a nonprofit organization have modified the bylaws to provide otherwise, each member is entitled to one vote.
- Members of nonprofit corporations do not have the right to sell their votes.
- Whenever a member makes a proper request, the organization's books or records of membership must be made available at either a regular meeting or a special meeting of the nonprofit corporation.
- A voting member may bring a court action to contest activities of a nonprofit organization that affect the member's rights or duties.

ARTICLES OF INCORPORATION

In Pennsylvania, the format and contents of Articles of Incorporation are governed by the Nonprofit Law which sets forth the specific provisions or requirements that must be met. When forming a nonprofit corporation, it is advisable to engage an attorney to review the law and assist in drafting the Articles. Articles of Incorporation must be filed with the Department of State. Generally, Articles of Incorporation must contain information including, but not limited to, the following:

- the name and registered address of the corporation;
- the purpose for which the organization was formed;
- a statement that the corporation is a not-for-profit corporation incorporated under the Nonprofit Corporation Law;
- the voting rights of members;
- the name and address of each individual incorporator;
- the effective date of the Articles; and
- whether or not the corporation is organized on a nonstock or a stock share basis.

BYLAWS

The bylaws of a nonprofit organization should be written carefully and clearly. Bylaws provide the framework for governance and management of the nonprofit organization. Bylaws regulate the conduct of all members of the nonprofit organization. Generally, bylaws dictate:

- the scope of the authority that has been granted to board members and members of senior management;
- the number of meetings that the organization must hold, the time period within which these meetings must occur (e.g., monthly, yearly, etc.), and the provisions for calling special meetings.

In certain instances, individuals or entities who do business with a nonprofit corporation and are aware of provisions within its bylaws may be subject to those provisions. Bylaws which are in clear opposition to Pennsylvania law will not be upheld.

SHARES OF STOCK IN A NONPROFIT CORPORATION

A nonprofit corporation may elect to have shareholders. If a nonprofit corporation chooses to have shareholders, the fact that the corporation is organized on a stock share basis must be clearly denoted in its Articles of Incorporation. The bylaws should describe the denominations in which shares will be issued and the shares should be evidenced by share certificates. The face of each share certificate must contain a conspicuous statement that the corporation for which it is issued is a nonprofit corporation.

Unless the bylaws state otherwise, holders are entitled to one vote per share. Similarly, unless the bylaws state otherwise, shares are nontransferable and may not be transferred by any method including operation of law. Shareholders are not entitled to and may not receive direct or indirect dividends on any shares. Further, shareholders of a charitable nonprofit corporation are not entitled to and may not receive any portion of the corporate earnings or corporate assets under any circumstance including its dissolution.

As long as the bylaws of a nonprofit corporation are lawful and reasonable, a shareholder who fails to comply with those bylaws may have their shares canceled by the nonprofit corporation and may be excluded from future membership.

CHARITABLE ASSETS

Property committed to charitable purposes has special protection under the law because it relieves the public burden by advancing one or more general or specific charitable causes. As soon as money or property is donated or committed to a charitable purpose, the Attorney General acts on behalf of the public's interest to ensure it is duly administered, including the assets held by nonprofit organizations formed for charitable purposes.

In Pennsylvania, the Orphans' Court has jurisdiction over property committed to charitable purposes under Rule 2156 of the Pennsylvania Rules of Judicial Administration, Pa. R.J.A. No. 2156, and under Section 711(21) of the Probate, Estates, and Fiduciaries Code, Act of July 1, 1972, *as amended,* 20 Pa. C.S.A. § 101-8815 (PEF Code), 20 Pa. C.S.A. § 711(21). The Nonprofit Law provides that charitable assets may not be diverted from the purposes for which they were donated, granted, or devised without obtaining an order from the Orphans' Court specifying the disposition of the assets, 15 Pa. C.S.A. §5547(b).

Under Rule 5.5 of the Supreme Court Orphans' Court Rules, the Attorney General must receive notice of any Orphans' Court proceeding involving or affecting charitable assets. Under the Commonwealth Attorneys Act, the Attorney General may intervene in any action involving charitable bequests or trusts, 71 P.S. §§ 732-101–732-208, §732-204(c). The termination of charitable trusts of $100,000 or less may be accomplished without an Orphans' Court proceeding if the Attorney General consents to it, 20 Pa. C.S.A. §7740.3(d).

Property committed to charitable purposes may be deemed to be held in trust regardless of whether a formal trust instrument has been prepared. If a trust instrument has been prepared, that document will govern investment and use of the assets or funds.

When a nonprofit organization is dissolved, the Orphans' Court must review the dissolution and approve the distribution of the assets.

A nonprofit corporation with responsibility for charitable assets acts as the trustee of those assets. Trustees are accountable for charitable assets and as such are responsible for ensuring that funds and assets are protected and invested wisely. A trustee that allows charitable assets to be squandered, diverted, or otherwise dissipated may be individually liable for the loss of those assets regardless of whether the assets were administered through a corporation.

CHARITABLE SOLICITATIONS

Most states, including Pennsylvania, regulate solicitations of charitable contributions. In Pennsylvania, charitable organizations and professional fundraisers are regulated by the Solicitation of Funds for Charitable Purposes Act, Act of December 19, 1990, P.L. 1200, *as amended*, 10 P.S. §§162.1–162.23 (Charities Act), and the Unfair Trade Practices and Consumer Protection Law, Act of December 17, 1968, P.L. 1224, *as amended*, 73 P.S. §§201-1–201-9.3 (Consumer Protection Law). In addition, certain fundraising activities such as Bingo and small games of chance are regulated at the state, local, and county levels.

Most charitable organizations and their fundraisers requesting donations within Pennsylvania are required to register with the

Department of State, Bureau of Charitable Organizations, prior to beginning any fundraising activities. Certain public service organizations and charitable organizations raising less than $25,000 annually are not required to register if they do not pay anyone to raise funds on their behalf. Even though a charitable organization may not be required to register before soliciting in Pennsylvania, these solicitations must still comply with all other provisions of the Charities Act and the Consumer Protection Law. The Charities Act requires that all charitable organizations "must establish and exercise control over fundraising activities conducted for its benefit, including approval of all written contracts and agreements, and must assure that fundraising activities are conducted without coercion." 10 P. S. §162.13(e).

Board members should also be aware that the Charities Act specifically states the standard of care that they must utilize in their treatment of property received as a result of a charitable solicitation. Section 21 holds that "every person soliciting, collecting or expending contributions for charitable purposes and every officer, director, trustee and employee of any such person concerned with the solicitation, collection, or expenditure of such contribution shall be deemed to be a *fiduciary* and acting in a *fiduciary capacity.*" 10 P. S. §162.21, (emphasis added).

To obtain registration forms and other information about registering a charitable organization or professional fundraiser contact the:

Commonwealth of Pennsylvania Department of State
Bureau of Charitable Organizations 207 North Office Building
Harrisburg, PA 17120
(717) 783–1720
(800) 732–0999
www.dos.state.pa.us/charity/index
(717) 783–1720
(800) 732–0999
www.dos.state.pa.us/charity/index

FUNDAMENTAL CHANGE TRANSACTIONS

The duties of the board of directors of a charitable nonprofit organization extend to all property committed to a charitable purpose. The Nonprofit Law provides that property committed to charitable purposes shall not "be diverted from the object to which it was donated, granted, or devised, unless and until the board of directors or other body obtains from the Court an order specifying the disposition of the property." 15 Pa. C.S.A. §5547 (b). The Probate, Estates, and Fiduciaries Code, Act of July 1, 1972, *as amended*, 20 Pa. C.S.A. § 101-8815 (PEF Code), has a similar requirement.

Whenever a nonprofit, charitable organization enters into a transaction effecting a fundamental corporate change that involves a transfer of ownership or control of all or substantially all of its charitable assets, the Office of Attorney General is obliged to review each transaction to ensure that the public interest is fully protected. These transactions may take various forms and include sales, mergers, consolidations, leases, options, conveyances, exchanges, transfers, joint ventures, affiliations, management agreements or collaboration arrangements, or other methods of disposition. The Office of Attorney General reviews such transactions regardless of whether the other party or parties to the transaction are nonprofit, mutual benefit or for-profit entities. Certain transactions that are in the usual and regular course of a nonprofit's activities will not be reviewed.

In December 1997, the Attorney General issued a Review Protocol for Fundamental Change Transactions Affecting Health Care Nonprofits to facilitate the review of nonprofit healthcare transactions. The Protocol was developed to be used as a guide by attorneys and staff in the Charitable Trusts and Organizations Section, and its outside experts, in reviewing fundamental change transactions affecting nonprofit, charitable health care entities. The principles underlying this protocol, however, are also applicable to non–health-care-related nonprofit corporations planning to undertake a fundamental change transaction.

To obtain a copy of the Protocol, please contact the Attorney General's Charitable Trusts and Organizations Section at the address below, or online at www.attorneygeneral.gov.

Office of Attorney General
Charitable Trusts and Organizations Section
14th Floor, Strawberry Square
Harrisburg, PA 17120
Telephone: 717–783-2853
www.attorneygeneral.gov
November 2011

SAMPLE MEMORANDUM OF AGREEMENT (RISK/PROFIT SHARING AGREEMENT FOR HEALTH CENTERS AND SOCIAL SERVICE PARTNERS)

MEMORANDUM OF AGREEMENT BETWEEN

Health Center Agency

&

Social Services Agency

This Memorandum of Agreement entered into as of *Date*, serves as a legally binding agreement (this "Agreement") between Health Center Agency and Social Services Agency (hereinafter collectively referred to as the "Parties"), concerning their roles and responsibilities regarding the Health Center Name or Grant #/HRSA Grant.

RECITALS

WHEREAS, Health Center Agency, EIN/Tax Id #, is *Brief Organization Description*; and

WHEREAS, Social Services Agency, EIN/Tax ID #, is *Brief Organization Description*.

WHEREAS, the Parties are working together to operate health care services at *health center sites (names/addresses)*. Health Center Name will serve *target population by name, population group (e.g., homeless)*; and

WHEREAS, the Parties wish to clearly define their roles and responsibilities with respect to the operation of the primary health care services to be provided at Health Center Name;

NOW THEREFORE, the Parties agree to the following:

1. The Parties will remain independent and separate entities.
2. The Parties intend to work together in the operation of Health Center Name in the following ways:
   a. Although Health Center Agency, as the Grant Award recipient, will be the formal operator of the Health Center Name

services to be provided through this Agreement, which will include, without limitation: primary health care, including HIV/AIDS treatment, behavioral health care, and related supplemental services such as pharmaceuticals, laboratory, diagnostic services, and certain additional services such as case management, outreach, advocacy, health promotion and education, and social work (the "Health Services"), Health Center Agency will consult on a regular basis with Social Services Agency regarding the Health Services. In consultation with Social Services Agency, Health Center Agency will be responsible for the clinical oversight of all primary health care, pharmaceutical, laboratory, diagnostic, and other services including clinical supervision of clinical staff, clinical services, collaborative physician agreements, and quality care. In consultation with Health Center Agency, Social Services Agency will be responsible for administrative oversight of functional aspects of service provision, including ensuring access and hours of operation. Hiring, discipline, and dismissal of primary care clinical staff and the hiring, discipline, and dismissal of other staff at Health Center Name will be discussed by both Health Center Agency and Social Services Agency. The final decisions regarding hiring, discipline, and dismissal will be made jointly by Health Center Agency Staff Designee and Social Services Agency Staff Designee. In consultation with Social Services Agency, Health Center Agency will be responsible for working to ensure that all required services and relationships are in place. As the operator of Health Center Name, all revenues will come to Health Center Agency, and the Parties will be reimbursed according to the mutually agreed upon budgets, with the understanding that program income and excess program income will be recognized consistent with program funding requirements. In consultation with Health Center Agency, Social Services Agency will be responsible for the day-to-day operation of behavioral health, case management, outreach, advocacy, health promotion and education, and social work services that will be provided to Health Center Name patients.

b. Between Health Center Agency and Social Services Agency, Social Services Agency will be the owner and lessee/subland-lord of all of the Health Center Agency facilities in which the Health Services will be provided and will be responsible for the physical layout, design, and outfitting said spaces to program funding standards, building maintenance and repair, and utilities. Social Services Agency is, and will remain, the owner of the name "Health Center Name" and in the event of the termination of this agreement, Health Center Agency will have no right to use the name "Health Center Name," or any version thereof, following the termination of this Agreement.

c. The Parties agree that all intellectual property that is created, discovered, or developed by Social Services Agency in connection with its provision of the services pursuant to this Agreement (including, without limitation, all such documents, reports, data management evaluation systems, and models of service) will be the sole and exclusive property of Social Services Agency, and Social Services Agency will be the sole and exclusive owner of any patents, trademarks, trade secrets, and copyrights in connection with said intellectual property, including, without limitation, the right to make application for statutory protection. All aforementioned information is hereinafter called "Social Services Agency Proprietary Information." Social Services Agency hereby grants to Health Center Agency a nonexclusive, non-sublicenseable, and nonassignable license to use any or all of the Social Services Agency Proprietary Information in connection with the operation of Health Center Name during the term of this Agreement. Further, all intellectual property that is created, discovered, or developed by Health Center Agency in connection with its provision of the services pursuant to this Agreement (including, without limitation, all such documents, reports, data management evaluation systems, and models of service) will be the sole and exclusive property of Health Center Agency, and Health Center Agency will be the sole and exclusive owner of any patents, trademarks, trade secrets, and copyrights in connection with said intellectual property, including, without limitation, the right to make application for statutory protection. All the aforementioned information is hereinafter called "Health Center Agency Proprietary Information." Health Center Agency hereby grants to Social Services Agency a nonexclusive, non-sublicenseable, and nonassignable license to use any or all of the Health Center Agency Proprietary Information in connection with the operation of Health Center Name during the term of this Agreement. All patients receiving services at Health Center Name will be treated as clients of Health Center Agency during the term of this Agreement.

d.   In consultation with Social Services Agency, Health Center Agency will be responsible for all central administrative functions of Health Center Name, such as billing, credentialing, etc., and will ensure that all requisite paperwork is complete, accurate, and timely. In consultation with Social Services Agency, Health Center Agency will provide electronic medical record and practice management technology and ensure that all staff involved have the training and ability to use such technology, including running reports.

e.   Social Services Agency will perform certain administrative operational functions of Health Center Name. The following provisions outline Health Center Agency's responsibility to Social Services Agency under this Agreement for costs relating to space, services, staffing, and administration.

   i.   *Space*: Social Services Agency will be the owner or lessee/sublandlord of all the facilities in which the Health Center Name sites operated in partnership with Social Services Agency will be located, and Social Services Agency will be responsible for the physical layout, design, and outfitting at said sites. Costs for space will be reimbursed in accordance with the mutually agreed upon budget in conjunction with the Grant Award.

   ii.   *Services*: Social Services Agency will provide behavioral health services, including drug and alcohol abuse counseling and treatment, that will be included in Health Center Name service mix. Social Services

Agency will be responsible for the day-to-day operation of these services under Health Center Agency oversight and supervision, and will report issues and concerns to Health Center Agency regarding clinical matters. Social Services Agency will be paid at a rate per service in accordance with the mutually agreed upon budget in conjunction with the Grant Award.

iii. *Staff and Administration*: Social Services Agency will provide certain staff who will participate in the operation of the health services, including social work, case management, outreach advocacy, health promotion and education services, and administration. While Social Services Agency will be responsible for the day-to-day supervision of these staff, these staff will come under the ultimate supervision of the CEO of Health Center Name, who must approve their selection to serve at Health Center Name and who can dismiss them from service at Health Center Name, all in consultation with the Social Services Agency Designee. Social Services Agency will bill Health Center Agency for the cost of these social work, case management, outreach, advocacy, health promotion and education services, and administrative staff. These costs will be reimbursed in accordance with the mutually agreed upon budget in conjunction with the Grant Award and in the manner set forth in 2a., above.

iv. *Billing and Reimbursement*: Social Services Agency will submit monthly to Health Center Agency all such documentation as may be required by HRSA to show and verify agreed upon reimbursable and reasonable costs relative to services provided by Social Services Agency under this Agreement during the prior month. Subject to the receipt of funds, Health Center Agency shall pay an amount equal to such costs so documented as are, in fact, paid by Social Services Agency and reimbursable or funded through the HRSA Grant Program, in a timely and reimbursable manner after receiving the required documentation, with such payments adjusted quarterly and at year end based upon the actual revenue/cost reconciliation. Health Center Agency will only reimburse based on a mutually agreed upon budget, including pre-approved salaries and expenses, and costs as provided in the foregoing sentence (it being agreed that such requirement is satisfied as to any item set forth in the Health Center's budget submitted to HRSA in conjunction with the Grant Award). Social Services Agency agrees that all outlays will comply with grant requirements and be reconciled to audited financial statements. This 2e.iv. will survive termination of this Agreement for any reason.

This Agreement complies with current Department of Health and Human Services (DHHS) policies and specifies without limitation:

1. *Quality of Services and Clinical Standards*: The Parties will continually monitor and strive to improve the quality of the care delivered to Health Center Agency patients. Social Services Agency will participate on the Health Center Agency continuous quality improvement committee (CQI) charged with monitoring the quality of service provided to Health Center Agency patients. This committee sets quality assurance standards and procedures. Social Services Agency will comply with the standards adopted by the CQI committee and will diligently monitor said compliance in a reasonable manner, and will take reasonable and prompt steps to correct any deficiencies. In the event of any such deficiencies, Social Services Agency will present a correction plan outlining the steps it will take to correct the deficiencies. Similarly, Health Center Agency will diligently monitor all of its clinical activities at Health Center Name, and in the event the CQI process identifies any deficiencies on the part of Health Center Agency, will work to present a correction plan outlining the steps it will take to correct the deficiencies.

2. *Liability Insurance*: Social Services Agency will maintain appropriate malpractice and general liability insurance in amounts mutually agreed upon by the Parties and shall provide proof of said insurance upon demand by Health Center Agency. Health Center Agency will reimburse such costs as provided for in the foregoing sentence in accordance with the mutually agreed upon budget submitted to HRSA in conjunction with the Grant Award. Health Center Agency and its staff, per FQHC guidelines, will be covered under the Federal Tort Claims Act, but will maintain general liability insurance in amounts mutually agreed by the Parties and will provide proof of said insurance upon demand by Social Services Agency.

3. *Procurement Standards*: Social Services Agency will comply with all applicable procurement standards or grant requirements, including conflict of interest standards.

4. *Maintenance of Medical Records*: Social Services Agency will establish the appropriate financial, program, and property management systems to maintain and store the medical records for Health Center Name patients. Health Center Agency will reimburse such costs as provided for in the foregoing sentence in accordance with the mutually agreed upon budget submitted to HRSA in conjunction with the Grant Award mentioned above. Social Services Agency will hold Health Center Name patient medical records in strict confidentiality in accordance with HIPAA requirements and the requirements of all state and federal privacy laws, regulations, and professional standards, including but not limited to 45 CFR Part 74. Social Services Agency and Health Center Agency will work collaboratively to determine options for data sharing as needed between Social Services Agency's and

Health Center Agency's data tracking systems. Social Services Agency will use the utmost care in the maintenance and storage of these Health Center Agency records. Health Center Agency and Social Services Agency will have full and unfettered access (including both physical access during normal business hours to paper-based records and electronic access to computerized records) to any and all of the medical records related to patients being served in connection with this Agreement, subject to the confidentiality of those records in accordance with applicable laws, regulations, and professional standards. In addition, DHHS and the U.S. Comptroller General will have access to patient records as required by law.

5.   *Advisory Board*: Health Center Agency and Social Services Agency will continue the functional community advisory committee that meets all of the requirements for a FQHC community board except those relating to governance authority and frequency of meeting, which have been waived as part of Health Center Agency's public housing special populations waiver. In terms of member composition, the community advisory committee must meet several requirements such as: (1) at least 9 but not more than 25 individuals, a majority of whom (51%) are users of Health Center Name; (2) fewer than half of the nonuser members shall be individuals who derive more than 10% of their annual income from the health care industry; and (3) the committee must be representative of the service area community, including from public housing, and have appropriate expertise in community affairs, local government, finance and banking, legal affairs, trade unions, and other commercial and industrial concerns, or social service agencies within the community. In order to meet these

requirements, this provision in no way limits or compromises the Health Center Agency Board's authority or limits its legislative and regulatory mandated functions and responsibilities.

f.   To enhance the operational relationship between Social Services Agency and Health Center Agency, representatives from both Parties who are part of the Health Center Name operations team will hold meetings at least monthly, involving leadership from each organization, at which time the Parties will discuss clinical, fiscal, budget, personnel, administrative, and planning matters as required in this Agreement. In the event of a difference of opinion between Social Services Agency and Health Center Agency, all reasonable efforts will be made by both Parties to ensure mutual cooperation and support while always promoting quality patient care. If Social Services Agency and Health Center Agency cannot agree after escalation of the issue to the leadership of both organizations, then either Party may seek mediation by a disinterested third party who is agreeable to both parties. In the event that HRSA provides a means for dispute resolution, either by statute or regulation, the Parties may agree to avail themselves of said means of dispute resolution in lieu of mediation. In the event of a breach of any provision of this agreement, the nonbreaching party shall provide notice to the breaching party of said breach, and the breaching party shall have thirty (30) days following the date of notice to cure said breach. If said breach is not cured within the time provided, either party may terminate this Agreement, after providing at least six (6) months advance written notice to the other Parties and to HRSA.

g.   The Parties agree to the following concerning their relationship:

   i.   *Solicitation of Former Employees*: The Parties agree that no party will solicit any employee formerly employed by another party to this Agreement for a period of one (1) year following the date on which that individual ceases his or her employment with the other party without first obtaining prior written consent from all parties involved. This provision will only apply to those employees who are included in the budgets for Health Center Name. This provision in no way limits or restricts the ability of the Parties to this Agreement to solicit, recruit, or hire persons contacted generally through the media, through recruiting firms, at career fairs, or through any other such means. Furthermore, this provision shall not survive the termination of this Agreement.

    ii.   *Marketing of Services*: The Parties will mutually agree on any articles, press releases, publications, or similar communications about Health Center Name, the relationship among the Parties, and the services offered at Health Center Name.

    iii.   *Independent Contractor Status*: The relationship of the Parties under this Agreement or any activity hereunder is as independent contractors only. This Agreement shall not be construed to establish a formal partnership, joint venture, or agency of any kind, and no party shall be considered the agent of, or have the authority to bind or incur indebtedness for, any other party.

3. The undertakings described in this Agreement will continue until the earlier of (a) six (6) months following the date on which Health Center Agency or Social Services Agency provides written notice to the other party of its intent to terminate this Agreement, (b) as provided in 2f. above, or (c) as provided in 2g. above.

4. Health Center Agency agrees not to submit any request to HRSA to renew the Grant Award or to open a new site of service within Social Services Agency's service area without Social Services Agency's prior written consent and approval, including a mutually agreed upon budget.

5. Each party will bear its own costs and expenses in connection with this Agreement except as described herein.

AGREED BY:

Health Center Agency Signatory   DATE

Social Services Agency Signatory   DATE

Index